PRAISE FOR
THE BUTCHERING ART

—

Short-listed for the 2018 Wellcome Book Prize

Short-listed for the 2018 Wolfson History Book Prize

An NPR Best Book of 2017

A *New York Times* Editors' Choice

An Ultimate BuzzFeed Books Gift Guide pick

A *Publishers Weekly* Book of the Week

A *Guardian* Book of the Day

—

"Vivid, gory." —Agatha French, *Los Angeles Times*

"[Fitzharris] paints a compelling portrait of a man of conviction, humour and, above all, humanity . . . *The Butchering Art* is thoroughly enjoyable." —Nicola Davis, *The Guardian*

"[A] vivid picture . . . Some of it reads as the brutal relic of a vanished past; some of it reads as a brutal relic of the present." —Genevieve Valentine, NPR

"Brilliant." —Kate Womersley, *The Spectator*

"With an eye for historical detail and an ear for vivid prose, Lindsey Fitzharris tells a spectacular story about one of the most important moments in the history of medicine: the rise of sterile surgery. *The Butchering Art* is a spectacular book—deliciously gruesome and utterly gripping. You will race through it, wincing as you go, but never wanting to stop."   —Ed Yong, bestselling author of
I Contain Multitudes

"*The Butchering Art* is medical history at its most visceral and vivid. It will make you forever grateful to Joseph Lister, the man who saved us from the horrors of pre-antiseptic surgery, and to Lindsey Fitzharris, who brings to life the harrowing and deadly sights, smells, and sounds of a nineteenth-century hospital."
—Caitlin Doughty, bestselling author of
Smoke Gets in Your Eyes and *From Here to Eternity*

"*The Butchering Art* is a brilliant account of the almost unimaginable horrors of surgery and postoperative infection before Joseph Lister transformed it all with his invention of antisepsis. It is the story of one of the truly great men of medicine and of the triumph of humane scientific method and dogged persistence over dogmatic ignorance."
—Henry Marsh, bestselling author of
Do No Harm and *Admissions*

"Electric. The drama of Lister's mission to shape modern medicine is as exciting as any novel."   —Dan Snow, BBC presenter and
author of *Battle Castles*

"Excellent . . . [Fitzharris] infuses her thoughtful and finely crafted examination of this [antiseptic] revolution with the same sense of wonder and compassion Lister himself brought to his patients, colleagues, and students . . . A remarkable life and time."
—*Publishers Weekly* (starred review)

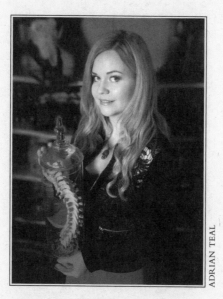

ADRIAN TEAL

LINDSEY FITZHARRIS

THE BUTCHERING ART

Lindsey Fitzharris received her PhD in the history of science and medicine from the University of Oxford. She is the creator of the popular website *The Chirurgeon's Apprentice*, and the writer and presenter of the YouTube series *Under the Knife*. She has written for *The Guardian*, *The Huffington Post*, *The Lancet*, and *New Scientist*. She lives in the English countryside with her husband, Adrian Teal, and their two cats. Visit her website at www.drlindsey fitzharris.com, follow her on Twitter at @DrLindseyFitz, and find her on Instagram at @drlindseyfitzharris.

THE BUTCHERING ART

JOSEPH LISTER'S QUEST

TO TRANSFORM THE GRISLY

WORLD OF VICTORIAN MEDICINE

THE
BUTCHERING ART

LINDSEY FITZHARRIS

SCIENTIFIC AMERICAN / FARRAR, STRAUS AND GIROUX

NEW YORK

Scientific American / Farrar, Straus and Giroux
175 Varick Street, New York 10014

An excerpt from *The Butchering Art* originally appeared,
in slightly different form, in *Scientific American*.

The Library of Congress has cataloged the hardcover edition as follows:
Names: Fitzharris, Lindsey, 1982– author.
Title: The butchering art / Lindsey Fitzharris.
Description: First edition. | New York : Scientific American / Farrar, Straus
    and Giroux, 2017. | Includes bibliographical references and index.
Identifiers: LCCN 2016059275 | ISBN 9780374117290 (hardcover) |
    ISBN 9780374715489 (ebook)
Subjects: LCSH: Lister, Joseph, Baron, 1827–1912. | Surgeons—Great
    Britain—Biography. | Surgery—Great Britain—History—19th century.
Classification: LCC RD27.35.L57 F58 2017 | DDC 617.092 [B]—dc23
LC record available at https://lccn.loc.gov/2016059275

Paperback ISBN: 978-0-374-53796-8

Designed by Richard Oriolo

Our books may be purchased in bulk for promotional, educational, or
business use. Please contact your local bookseller or the Macmillan Corporate
and Premium Sales Department at 1-800-221-7945, extension 5442, or
by e-mail at MacmillanSpecialMarkets@macmillan.com.

www.fsgbooks.com • books.scientificamerican.com
www.twitter.com/fsgbooks • www.facebook.com/fsgbooks

Scientific American is a registered trademark of Nature America, Inc.

9   10

FRONTISPIECE: Artist/maker unknown. After Thomas Eakins,
The Agnew Clinic. c. 1889. Photogravure.
(Philadelphia Museum of Art, Gift of Samuel B. Sturgis, 1973-268-190)

To my grandma Dorothy Sissors,

my bonus in life

CONTENTS

THE BUTCHERING ART

PROLOGUE:
THE AGE OF AGONY

—

**When a distinguished but elderly scientist states that
something is possible, he is almost certainly right.
When he states that something is impossible,
he is almost certainly wrong.**

—ARTHUR C. CLARKE

ON THE AFTERNOON OF DECEMBER 21, 1846, hundreds of men crowded into the operating theater at London's University College Hospital, where the city's most renowned surgeon was preparing to enthrall them with a mid-thigh amputation. As the people filed in, they were entirely unaware that they were about to witness one of the most pivotal moments in the history of medicine.

The theater was filled to the rafters with medical students and curious spectators, many of whom had dragged in with them the dirt and grime of everyday life in Victorian London. The surgeon John Flint South remarked that the rush and scuffle to get a place in an operating theater was not unlike that for a seat in the pit or gallery of a playhouse. People were packed like herrings in a basket, with those in the back rows constantly jostling for a better view, shouting out "Heads, heads" whenever their line of sight was blocked. At times, the floor of a theater like this one could be so crowded that the surgeon couldn't operate until it had been partially cleared. Even though it was December, the atmosphere inside the theater was stifling, verging on unbearable. The crush of bodies made the place feel plaguey hot.

The audience was made up of an eclectic group of men, some of whom were neither medical professionals nor students. The first two rows of an operating theater were typically occupied by "hospital dressers," a term that referred to those who accompanied surgeons on their rounds, carrying boxes of supplies needed to dress wounds. Behind the dressers stood the pupils, who restlessly pushed and murmured to one another in the back rows, as well as honored guests and other members of the public.

Medical voyeurism was nothing new. It arose in the dimly lit anatomical amphitheaters of the Renaissance, where, in front of transfixed spectators, the bodies of executed criminals were dissected as an additional punishment for their crimes. Ticketed spectators watched anatomists slice into the distended bellies of decomposing corpses, parts gushing forth not only human blood but also fetid pus. The lilting but incongruous notes of a flute sometimes accompanied the macabre demonstration. Public dissections were *theatrical* performances, a form of entertainment as popular as cockfighting or bearbaiting. Not everyone had the stomach for it, though. The French philosopher Jean-Jacques Rousseau said of the experience, "What a terrible sight an anatomy theatre is! Stinking corpses, livid running flesh, blood, repellent intestines, horrible skeletons, pestilential vapors! Believe me, this is not the place where [I] will go looking for amusement."

The operating theater at University College Hospital looked more or less the same as others in the city. It consisted of a stage partially enclosed by semicircular stands rising one above another toward a large skylight that illuminated the area below. On days when swollen clouds blotted out the sun, thick candles lit the scene. In the middle of the room was a wooden table stained with the telltale signs of past butcheries. Underneath it, the floor was strewn with sawdust to soak up the blood that would shortly issue from the severed limb. On most days, the screams of those struggling under the knife mingled discordantly with everyday noises drifting in from the street below: children laughing, people chatting, carriages rumbling by.

In the 1840s, operative surgery was a filthy business fraught with hidden dangers. It was to be avoided at all costs. Due to the risks, many surgeons refused to operate altogether, choosing instead to limit their scope to the treatment of external ailments like skin conditions and superficial wounds. Invasive procedures were few and far between, which was one of the reasons why so many spectators flocked to the operating theater on the day of a procedure. In 1840, for instance, only 120 operations were performed at Glasgow's Royal Infirmary. Surgery was always a last resort and only done in matters of life and death.

The physician Thomas Percival advised surgeons to change their aprons and to clean the table and instruments between procedures, not for hygienic purposes, but to avoid "every thing that may incite terror." Few heeded his advice. The surgeon, wearing a blood-encrusted apron, rarely washed his hands or his instruments and carried with him into the theater the unmistakable smell of rotting flesh, which those in the profession cheerfully referred to as "good old hospital stink."

At a time when surgeons believed pus was a natural part of the healing process rather than a sinister sign of sepsis, most deaths were due to postoperative infections. Operating theaters were gateways to death. It was safer to have an operation at home than in a hospital, where mortality rates were three to five times higher than they were in domestic settings. As late as 1863, Florence Nightingale declared, "The actual mortality in hospitals, especially in those of large crowded cities, is very much higher than any calculation founded on the mortality of the same class of diseases amongst patients treated out of the hospital would lead us to expect." Being treated at home, however, was expensive.

The infections and the filth weren't the only problems. Surgery was painful. For centuries, people sought ways to make it less so. Although nitrous oxide had been recognized as a painkiller since the chemist Joseph Priestley first synthesized it in 1772, "laughing gas" was not normally used in surgery, because its results were unreliable. Mesmerism—named after the German physician Franz Anton Mesmer, who invented the hypnotic technique in the 1770s—had also failed to be accepted into mainstream medical practice in the eighteenth century. Mesmer and his followers thought that when they moved their hands in front of patients, a physical influence of some kind was generated over them. This influence created positive physiological changes that would help patients heal and could also imbue a person with psychic powers. Most doctors remained unconvinced.

Mesmerism enjoyed a brief revival in Britain in the 1830s, when the physician John Elliotson began holding public displays at University College Hospital during which two of his patients, Elizabeth and Jane O'Key, were able to predict the fate of other hospital patients. Under Elliotson's hypnotic influence, they claimed to see "Big Jacky" (otherwise known as Death) hovering over the beds of those who later died. Any serious interest in Elliotson's methods was short-lived, however. In 1838, the editor of *The Lancet*, the world's leading medical journal, tricked the O'Key sisters into confessing their fraud, thus exposing Elliotson as a charlatan.

The scandal was still fresh in the minds of those attending University College Hospital on the afternoon of December 21, when the renowned surgeon Robert Liston announced he'd be testing the efficacy of ether on his patient. "We are going to try a Yankee dodge today, gentlemen, for making men insensible!" he declared as he made his way to the center of the stage. A hush fell over the theater as he began to speak. Like mesmerism, the use of ether was seen as a suspect foreign technique for putting people into a subdued state of consciousness. It was referred to as the Yankee dodge due to its being first used as a general anesthetic in America. It had been discovered in 1275, but its stupefying effects weren't synthesized until 1540, when the German botanist and chemist Valerius Cordus created a revolutionary formula that involved adding sulfuric acid to ethyl alcohol. His contemporary Paracelsus experimented with ether on chickens, noting that when the birds drank the liquid, they would undergo prolonged sleep and awake unharmed. He concluded that the substance "quiets all suffering without any harm and relieves all pain, and quenches all fevers, and prevents complications in all disease." Yet it would be several hundred years before it was tested on humans.

That moment came in 1842, when Crawford Williamson Long became the first documented doctor to use ether as a general anesthetic, in an operation to remove a tumor from a patient's neck in Jefferson, Georgia. Unfortunately, Long didn't publish the results of his experiments until 1848. By that time, the Boston dentist William T. G. Morton had won fame in September 1846 by using ether on a patient while extracting a tooth. An account of this successful and painless procedure was published in a newspaper, prompting a notable surgeon to ask Morton to assist him in an operation removing a large tumor from a patient's lower jaw at Massachusetts General Hospital.

On November 18, 1846, Dr. Henry Jacob Bigelow wrote about

this groundbreaking moment in *The Boston Medical and Surgical Journal*: "It has long been an important problem in medical science to devise some method of mitigating the pain of surgical operations. An efficient agent for this purpose has at length been discovered." Bigelow went on to describe how Morton had administered what he called "Letheon" to the patient before the operation commenced. This was a gas named after the river Lethe in classical mythology, which made the souls of the dead forget their lives on earth. Morton, who had patented the composition of the gas shortly after the operation, kept its parts secret, even from the surgeons. Bigelow revealed, however, that he could detect the sickly sweet smell of ether in it. News about the miraculous substance that could render people unconscious during surgery spread quickly around the world as surgeons rushed to test the effects of ether on their own patients.

Back in London, the American physician Francis Boott received a letter from Bigelow giving a full account of the momentous events in Boston. Intrigued, Boott persuaded the dental surgeon James Robinson to administer ether during one of his many tooth extractions. The experiment was such a success that Boott hurried over to University College Hospital to speak to Robert Liston that very same day.

Liston was skeptical, though not enough to pass up an opportunity to try something new in the operating theater. If nothing else, it would make for a good show, something for which he was known throughout the country. He agreed to use it in his next operation, scheduled two days hence.

Liston arrived on the scene in London at a time when "gentleman physicians" held considerable power and influence over the medical community. They were part of the ruling elite, forming the top of a medical pyramid. As such, they acted as gatekeepers for their

profession, admitting only men whom they believed had good breeding and high moral standing. They themselves were bookish types
with very little practical training who used their minds, not their
hands, to treat patients. Their education was rooted in the classics. It
was not uncommon during this period for physicians to prescribe
treatment without first performing a physical examination. Indeed,
some dispensed medical advice through letters alone, never laying
eyes on the patient in question.

In contrast, surgeons came from a long tradition of being trained
through apprenticeships, the value of which depended heavily on
the master's capabilities. Theirs was a practical trade, one to be taught
by precept and example. Many surgeons in the first decades of the
nineteenth century didn't attend university. Some were even illiterate.
Directly below them were the apothecaries, who were in charge of
dispensing drugs. In theory, there was a clear demarcation between
the surgeon and the apothecary. In practice, a man who had been
apprenticed to a surgeon might also act as an apothecary and vice
versa. This gave rise to an unofficial fourth category, the "surgeon-
apothecary," who was akin to the modern general practitioner. The
surgeon-apothecary was a doctor of first resort for the poor, especially
outside London.

Beginning in 1815, a form of systematic education began to
emerge in the medical world, driven in part by a broader demand
within the country for uniformity in a fragmented system. For
surgical students in London, reform brought about requirements
that they attend lectures and walk the wards of hospitals for at least
six months before obtaining a license from the profession's governing body, the Royal College of Surgeons. Teaching hospitals
began to spring up all over the capital, the first appearing at Charing Cross in 1821, with University College Hospital and King's
College Hospital following in 1834 and 1839, respectively. If one
wanted to go a step further and become a member of the Royal

College of Surgeons, he had to spend at least six years in professional study, including three years at a hospital; submit written accounts of at least six clinical cases; and take a grueling two-day examination that sometimes required him to perform dissections and operations on a cadaver.

The surgeon thus began his evolution from an ill-trained technician to a modern surgical specialist in those first decades of the nineteenth century. As an instructor at one of the newly built teaching hospitals in London, Robert Liston was very much a part of this ongoing transformation.

At six feet two, Liston was eight inches taller than the average British male. He had built his reputation on brute force and speed at a time when both were crucial to the survival of the patient. Those who came to witness an operation might miss it if they looked away even for a moment. It was said of Liston by his colleagues that when he amputated, "the gleam of his knife was followed so instantaneously by the sound of sawing as to make the two actions appear almost simultaneous." His left arm was reportedly so strong that he could use it as a tourniquet, while he wielded the knife in his right hand. This was a feat that required immense strength and dexterity, given that patients often struggled against the fear and agony of the surgeon's assault. Liston could remove a leg in less than thirty seconds, and in order to keep both hands free, he often clasped the bloody knife between his teeth while working.

Liston's speed was both a gift and a curse. Once, he accidentally sliced off a patient's testicle along with the leg he was amputating. His most famous (and possibly apocryphal) mishap involved an operation during which he worked so rapidly that he took off three of his assistant's fingers and, while switching blades, slashed a spectator's coat. Both the assistant and the patient died later of gangrene, and the unfortunate bystander expired on the spot from fright. It is the only surgery in history said to have had a 300 percent fatality rate.

Indeed, the perils of shock and pain limited surgical treatments before the dawn of anesthetics. One surgical text from the eighteenth century declared, "Painful methods are always the last remedies in the hands of a man that is truly able in his profession; and they are the first, or rather they are the only resource of him whose knowledge is confined to the art of operating." Those desperate enough to go under the knife were subject to unimaginable agony.

The traumas of the operating theater could take a toll on student spectators too. The Scottish obstetrician James Y. Simpson fled an amputation of the breast when he was studying at the University of Edinburgh. The sight of the soft tissues being lifted with a hook-like instrument and the surgeon preparing to make two sweeping cuts around the breast proved too much for Simpson. He forced his way back through the crowd, exited the theater, hurried through the hospital gates, and made his way up to Parliament Square, where he declared breathlessly that he now wished to study law. Fortunately for posterity, Simpson—who would go on to discover chloroform—was dissuaded from pursuing a change of career.

Although Liston was all too aware of what awaited his patients on the operating table, he often downplayed the horrors for the sake of protecting their nerves. Just months before his experiment with ether, he removed the leg of a twelve-year-old child named Henry Pace, who had been suffering from a tubercular swelling of the right knee. The boy asked the surgeon whether the operation would hurt, and Liston responded, "No more than having a tooth out." When the moment came to have his leg removed, Pace was brought into the theater blindfolded and pinned down by Liston's assistants. The boy counted six strokes of the saw before his leg dropped off. Sixty years later, Pace would recount the story to medical students at University College London—the horror of the experience, no doubt, fresh in his mind as he sat in the very hospital in which he had lost his leg.

Like many surgeons operating in a pre-anesthetic era, Liston had learned to steel himself against the cries and protests of those strapped to the blood-spattered operating table. On one occasion, Liston's patient, who had come in to have a bladder stone removed, ran from the room in terror and locked himself in the lavatory before the procedure could begin. Liston, hot on his heels, broke the door down and dragged the screaming patient back to the operating room. There, he bound the man fast before passing a curved metal tube up the patient's penis and into the bladder. He then slid a finger into the man's rectum, feeling for the stone. Once Liston had located it, his assistant removed the metal tube and replaced it with a wooden staff, which acted as a guide so the surgeon wouldn't fatally rupture the patient's rectum or intestines as he began cutting deep into the bladder. Once the staff was in place, Liston cut diagonally through the fibrous muscle of the scrotum until he reached the wooden staff. Next, he used the probe to widen the hole, ripping open the prostate gland in the process. At this point, he removed the wooden staff and used forceps to extract the stone from the bladder.

Liston—who reportedly had the fastest knife in the West End—achieved all this in just under sixty seconds.

—

NOW, AS LISTON stood before those gathered in the new operating theater of University College London a few days before Christmas, the veteran surgeon held in his hands the jar of clear liquid ether that might do away with the need for speed in surgery. If it lived up to American claims, the nature of surgery might change forever. Still, Liston couldn't help wondering whether the ether was just another product of quackery that would have little or no useful application in surgery.

Tensions were high. Just fifteen minutes before Liston entered the theater, his colleague William Squire had turned to the packed crowd of onlookers and asked for a volunteer to practice on. A nervous murmur filled the room. In Squire's hand was an apparatus that looked like an Arabian hookah made of glass with a rubber tube and bell-shaped mask. The device had been fashioned by Squire's uncle, a pharmacist in London, and used by the dental surgeon James Robinson to extract a tooth just two days prior. It looked foreign to those in the audience. None dared to have it tested on them.

Exasperated, Squire ordered the theater's porter Shelldrake to submit to the trial. He wasn't a good choice, because he was "fat, plethoric, and with a liver no doubt very used to strong liquor." Squire gently placed the apparatus over the man's fleshy face. After a few deep breaths of ether, the porter reportedly leaped off the table and ran out of the room, cursing the surgeon and crowd at the top of his lungs.

There would be no more tests. The unavoidable moment had arrived.

At twenty-five minutes past two in the afternoon, Frederick Churchill—a thirty-six-year-old butler from Harley Street—was brought in on a stretcher. The young man had been suffering from chronic osteomyelitis of the tibia, a bacterial bone infection which had caused his right knee to swell and become violently bent. His first operation came three years earlier, when the inflamed area was opened up and "a number of irregularly shaped laminated bodies" ranging from the size of a pea to that of a large bean were removed. On November 23, 1846, Churchill was once again back in the hospital. A few days later, Liston made an incision and passed a probe into the knee. Using his unwashed hands, Liston felt for the bone to ensure it wasn't loose. He ordered that the opening be washed with warm water and dressed and that the patient be allowed to rest. Over the next few days, however, Churchill's condition deteriorated. He soon experienced sharp pain that radiated from his hip to his toes. This occurred again three weeks later, after which Liston decided the leg must come off.

Churchill was carried into the operating theater on a stretcher and laid out on the wooden table. Two assistants stood nearby in case the ether did not take effect and they had to resort to restraining the terrified patient while Liston removed the limb. At Liston's signal, Squire stepped forward and held the mask over Churchill's mouth. Within a few minutes, the patient was unconscious. Squire then placed an ether-soaked handkerchief over Churchill's face to ensure he wouldn't wake during the operation. He nodded to Liston and said, "I think he will do, sir."

Liston opened a long case and removed a straight amputation knife of his own invention. An observer in the audience that afternoon noted that the instrument must have been a favorite, for on the handle were little notches showing the number of times he had used it before. Liston grazed his thumbnail over the blade to test its sharpness. Satisfied that it would do the job, he instructed his assistant William Cadge to "take the artery" and then turned to the crowd.

"Now, gentlemen, time me!" he yelled. A ripple of clicks rang out as pocket watches were pulled from waistcoats and flipped open.

Liston turned back to the patient and clamped his left hand around the man's thigh. In one rapid movement, he made a deep incision above the right knee. One of his assistants immediately tightened a tourniquet around the leg to halt the flow of blood while Liston pushed his fingers up underneath the flap of skin to pull it back. The surgeon made another series of quick maneuvers with his knife, exposing the thighbone. He then paused.

Many surgeons, once confronted with exposed bone, felt daunted by the task of sawing through it. Earlier in the century, Charles Bell cautioned students to saw slowly and deliberately. Even those who were adept at making incisions could lose their nerve when it came to cutting off a limb. In 1823, Thomas Alcock proclaimed that humanity "shudders at the thought, that men unskilled in any other tools than the daily use of the knife and fork, should with unhallowed hands presume to operate upon their suffering fellow-creatures." He recalled a spine-chilling story about a surgeon whose saw became so tightly wedged in the bone that it wouldn't budge. His contemporary William Gibson advised that novices practice with a piece of wood to avoid such nightmarish scenarios.

Liston handed the knife to one of the surgical dressers, who, in return, handed him a saw. The same assistant drew up the muscles, which would later be used in forming an adequate stump for the amputee. The great surgeon made half a dozen strokes before the limb fell off, into the waiting hands of a second assistant, who promptly tossed it into a box full of sawdust just to the side of the operating table.

Meanwhile, the first assistant momentarily released the tourniquet to reveal the severed arteries and veins that would need to be tied up. In a mid-thigh amputation, there are commonly eleven to secure by ligature. Liston tied off the main artery with a square knot and then turned his attention to the smaller blood vessels, which he drew up one by one using a sharp hook called a tenaculum. His assistant loosened the tourniquet once more while Liston stitched the remaining flesh closed.

It took all of twenty-eight seconds for Liston to remove Churchill's right leg, during which time the patient neither stirred nor cried out. When the young man awoke a few minutes later, he reportedly asked when the surgery would begin and was answered by the sight of his elevated stump, much to the amusement of the spectators who sat astounded by what they had just witnessed. His face alight with the excitement of the moment, Liston announced, "This Yankee dodge, gentlemen, beats mesmerism hollow!"

The age of agony was nearing its end.

—

TWO DAYS LATER, the surgeon James Miller read a hastily penned letter from Liston to his medical students in Edinburgh, "announcing in enthusiastic terms, that a new light had burst on Surgery." During the first few months of 1847, both surgeons and curious celebrities visited operating theaters to witness the miracle of ether. Everyone from Sir Charles Napier, colonial governor of what is now a province of Pakistan, to Prince Jérôme Bonaparte, the youngest brother of Napoleon I, came to see the effects of ether with their own eyes.

The term "etherization" was coined, and its use in surgery was celebrated in newspapers around the country. News of its powers spread. "The history of Medicine has presented no parallel to the perfect success that has attended the use of ether," the *Exeter Flying Post* proclaimed. Liston's success was also trumpeted in the London *People's Journal*: "Oh, what delight for every feeling heart . . . the announcement of this noble discovery of the power to still the sense of pain, and veil the eye and memory from all the horrors of an operation. . . . WE HAVE CONQUERED PAIN!"

Equally momentous to Liston's triumph with ether was the presence that day of a young man named Joseph Lister, who had seated himself quietly at the back of the operating theater. Dazzled and enthralled by the dramatic performance, this aspiring medical student realized as he walked out of the theater onto Gower Street that the nature of his future profession would forever be changed. No longer would he and his classmates have to behold "so horrible and distressing a scene" as that observed by William Wilde, a surgical student who was reluctantly present at the excision of a patient's eyeball without anesthetic. Nor would they feel the need to escape, as John Flint South had done whenever the cries of those being butchered by a surgeon grew intolerable.

Nevertheless, as Lister made his way through the crowds of men shaking hands and congratulating themselves on their choice of profession and this notable victory, he was acutely aware that pain was only one impediment to successful surgery.

He knew that for thousands of years, the ever-looming threat of infection had restricted the extent of a surgeon's reach. Entering the abdomen, for instance, had proven almost uniformly fatal because of it. The chest was also off-limits. For the most part, whereas physicians treated internal conditions—hence the term "internal medicine," which still persists today—surgeons dealt with peripheral ones: lacerations, fractures, skin ulcers, burns. Only with amputations did the surgeon's knife penetrate deep into the body. Surviving the operation was one thing. Making a full recovery was another.

As it turned out, the two decades immediately following the popularization of anesthesia saw surgical outcomes worsen. With their newfound confidence about operating without inflicting pain, surgeons became ever more willing to take up the knife, driving up the incidences of postoperative infection and shock. Operating theaters became filthier than ever as the number of surgeries increased. Surgeons still lacking an understanding of the causes of infection would operate on multiple patients in succession using the same unwashed instruments on each occasion. The more crowded the operating theater became, the less likely it was that even the most primitive sanitary precautions would be taken. Of those who went under the knife, many either died or never fully recovered and then spent the rest of their lives as invalids. This problem was universal. Patients worldwide came to further dread the word "hospital," while the most skilled surgeons distrusted their own abilities.

With Robert Liston's ether triumph, Lister had just witnessed the elimination of the first of the two major obstacles to successful surgery—that it could now be performed without inflicting pain.

Inspired by what he had seen on the afternoon of December 21, the deeply perceptive Joseph Lister would soon embark on devoting the rest of his life to elucidating the causes and nature of postoperative infections and finding a solution for them. In the shadow of one of the profession's last great butchers, another surgical revolution was about to begin.

1.

THROUGH THE LENS

—

Let us not overlook the further great fact, that not
only does science underlie sculpture, painting, music,
poetry, but that science is itself poetic. . . . Those
engaged in scientific researches constantly show us that
they realize not less vividly, but more vividly,
than others, the poetry of their subjects.

—HERBERT SPENCER

LITTLE JOSEPH LISTER STOOD ON his toes and put his eye to the ocular lens of his father's latest compound microscope. Unlike the foldaway versions that tourists tucked in their pockets and carried with them on trips to the seaside, the instrument before him was something altogether grander. It was sleek, handsome, powerful: a symbol of scientific progress.

The very first time he looked down the barrel of a microscope, Lister marveled at the intricate world that had previously been hidden from his sight. He delighted in the fact that the objects he could observe under the magnifying lens were seemingly infinite. Once, he plucked a shrimp from the sea and watched in awe at "the heart beating very rapidly" and "the aorta pulsating." He noticed how the blood slowly circulated through the surface of the limbs and over the back of the heart as the creature wriggled under his gaze.

Lister was born on April 5, 1827, to no fanfare. Six months later, though, his mother gushed to her husband in a letter, "The baby has been today unusually lovely." He was the couple's fourth child and second son, one of seven children to be born to Joseph Jackson Lister and his wife, Isabella, two devout Quakers.

Lister had plenty of opportunities to explore miniature worlds with the microscope while he was growing up. Simplicity was the Quaker way of life. Lister wasn't allowed to hunt, participate in sports, or attend the theater. Life was a gift to be employed in honoring God and helping one's neighbor, not in the pursuit of frivolities. Because of this, many Quakers turned to scientific endeavors, one of the few pastimes allowed by their faith. It was not uncommon to find among those even in modest circumstances an intellectual man of high scientific attainments.

Lister's father exemplified this. At the age of fourteen, he left school and became an apprentice to his own father, a wine merchant. Although many Quakers abstained from consuming alcohol in the Victorian period, their faith did not explicitly forbid it. The Lister family's business was centuries old, begun at a time when teetotalism among Quakers hadn't yet gained popularity. Joseph Jackson became a partner in his father's wine business, but it was his discoveries in optics that would earn him worldwide renown during Lister's childhood. He had first become interested in the subject as a young boy when he discovered that a bubble trapped in the window glass of his own father's study acted as a simple magnifier.

At the beginning of the nineteenth century, most microscopes were sold as gentlemen's toys. They were housed in expensive cases lined with plush velvet. Some were mounted on square wooden bases that contained accessory drawers holding extra lenses, rods, and fittings that more often than not went unused. Most makers supplied their wealthy clients with a set of prepared slides of animal bone sections, fish scales, and delicate flowers. Very few people who purchased a microscope during this period did so for serious scientific purposes.

Joseph Jackson Lister was an exception. Between 1824 and 1843, he became a great devotee of the instrument and set out to correct many of its defects. Most lenses caused distortion due to light of different wavelengths being diffracted at various angles through glass. This produced a purple halo around the object in view: an effect that led many to distrust the microscope's revelations. Joseph Jackson toiled to fix this flaw and in 1830 showcased his achromatic lens, which eliminated the distracting halo. While engaged with his own business, Joseph Jackson somehow found time to grind lenses himself and supply the mathematical calculations necessary for their manufacture to some of the leading makers of microscopes in London. His work earned him a fellowship in the Royal Society in 1832.

On the first floor of little Lister's childhood home was the "museum," a room filled with hundreds of fossils and other specimens that various members of the family had collected over the years. His father insisted that each of his children read to him in the mornings while he dressed. Their library consisted of a collection of religious and scientific tomes. One of Joseph Jackson's earliest gifts to his son was a four-volume book called *Evenings at Home; or, The Juvenile Budget Opened*, which contained fables, fairy tales, and natural history.

Lister escaped many of the dangerous medical treatments that some of his contemporaries experienced while growing up, because his father believed in *vis medicatrix naturae*, or "the healing power of nature." Like many Quakers, Joseph Jackson was a therapeutic nihilist, adhering to the idea that Providence played the most important role in the healing process. He believed that administering foreign substances to the body was unnecessary and sometimes downright life-threatening. In an age when most medicinal concoctions contained highly toxic drugs like mercury and arsenic, Joseph Jackson's ideas might not have been too wide of the mark.

Because of the household's dearly held principles, it came as a surprise to everyone in the family when young Lister announced that he wanted to be a surgeon—a job that involved physically intervening in God's handiwork. None of his relations, except a distant cousin, were doctors. And surgery, in particular, carried with it a certain social stigma even for those outside the Quaker community. The surgeon was very much viewed as a manual laborer who used his hands to make his living, much like a key cutter or plumber today. Nothing better demonstrated the inferiority of surgeons than their relative poverty. Before 1848, no major hospital had a salaried surgeon on its staff, and most surgeons (with the exception of a notable few) made very little money from their private practices.

But the impact a medical career might have on his social and financial standing later in life was far from Lister's mind when he was a boy. During the summer of 1841, at the age of fourteen, he wrote to his father, who was away attending to the family's wine business, "When Mamma was out I was by myself and had nothing to do but draw skeletons." Lister requested a sable brush so that he could "shade another man to shew the rest of the muscles." He drew and labeled all the bones in the cranium, as well as those of the hands, from both the front and the back. Like his father, young Lister was a proficient artist—a skill that would later help him to document in startling detail his observations made during his medical career.

Lister was also preoccupied with a sheep's head that summer of 1841 and in the same letter declared, "I got almost all the meat off; and I think all the brains out . . . [before] putting it into the macerating tub." He did this to soften the remaining tissue on the skull. Later, he had managed to articulate the skeleton of a frog he had dissected after stealing a piece of wood from his sister's cabinet drawer onto which he anchored the creature. He wrote to his father with glee, "It looks just as if [the frog] was going to take a leap," adding, conspiratorially, "Do not tell Mary about the piece of wood."

Whatever Joseph Jackson Lister's reservations were about the medical profession, it was clear that his son would soon be joining its professional ranks.

LISTER FOUND HIMSELF very far away from the life he had known as a child when he began his studies at University College London (UCL) at the age of seventeen. His village of Upton was small by comparison, with 12,738 inhabitants. Although only ten miles from the city, Upton could only be reached by horse and buggy trundling along the muddy tracks that passed for roads at that time. An oriental bridge crossed a stream that flowed through the Listers' garden, in which there were apple, beech, elm, and chestnut trees. His father wrote of the "folding windows open to the garden; and the temperate warmth and stillness, and the chirping of birds and hum of insects, the bright lawn and aloe and the darker spread of the cedars and chequered sky above."

In contrast to the vivid colors of the lush gardens surrounding Upton House, London was blocked out in a palette of gray. The art critic John Ruskin called it a "ghastly heap of fermenting brickwork, pouring out poison at every pore." Garbage was habitually heaped outside houses, some of which had no doors because the poor often used them as fuel for their grates during the winter months. Roads and alleyways were soiled with manure from the thousands of saddled horses, carts, omnibuses, and hansom cabs that rattled through the city each day. Everything—from the buildings to the people—was covered in a layer of soot.

Within the space of a hundred years, London's population soared from one million to just over six million inhabitants in the nineteenth century. The wealthy left the city in search of greener pastures, leaving behind grand homes that soon fell into disrepair as they were appropriated by the masses. Single rooms might contain thirty or more people of all ages clad in soiled rags and squatting, sleeping, and defecating in straw-filled billets. The extremely poor were forced to live in "cellar homes," permanently shut off from sunlight. The rats gnawed at the faces and fingers of malnourished infants, many of whom died in these dark, fetid, and damp surroundings.

Death was a frequent visitor to London's inhabitants, and disposing of the deceased was a growing problem. Churchyards were bursting at the seams with human remains, posing huge threats to public health. It was not uncommon to see bones projecting from freshly turned ground. Bodies were crammed on top of one another in graves, most of which were merely open pits with row after row of coffins. At the beginning of the century, two men purportedly asphyxiated on gases emanating from decomposing bodies after they fell twenty feet to the bottom of a burial pit.

For those living near these pits, the smell was unbearable. The houses on Clement's Lane in East London backed onto the local churchyard, which oozed with putrid slime; the stench was so overpowering that occupants kept their windows shut all year long. Children attending the local Sunday school at Enon Chapel could not escape this unpleasantness. They were given their lessons as flies buzzed around them, no doubt originating from inside the church's crypt, which was stuffed with twelve thousand rotting corpses.

Arrangements for the disposal of human waste were equally rudimentary before the passing of the Public Health Act in 1848, which established the centralized General Board of Health and initiated a sanitarian revolution. Before then, many streets in London were effectively open sewers, releasing powerful (and often deadly) amounts of methane. In the worst housing developments, lines of domiciles known as "back-to-backs" were separated only by narrow passageways four to five feet wide. Trenches brimming with piss ran down the middle. Even the increased number of water closets between 1824 and 1844 did little to solve the problem. Their construction forced landlords to hire men to remove "night soil" from overflowing cesspools in the city's buildings. An entire underground army of "bone boilers," "toshers," and "mud-larks" developed to exploit the tide of human waste underneath the city. These scavengers—whom the author Steven Johnson calls history's first waste recyclers—would pick through the thousands of pounds of garbage, feces, and animal corpses and then cart off these foul goods to market, where they could be reused by tanners, farmers, and other traders.

The business conducted elsewhere wasn't any more wholesome. Fat boilers, glue renderers, fellmongers, tripe scrapers, and dog skinners all went about their malodorous tasks in some of the most densely populated areas of the city. For instance, in Smithfield—just a few minutes' walk from St. Paul's Cathedral—was a slaughterhouse. Its walls were caked with putrefied blood and fat. Sheep were hurled into its depths, breaking their legs before being knifed, flayed, and butchered by the men below. After a long day's work, these same men carried on their clothes the ordure of their unholy profession back to the slums in which they lived.

This was a world crawling with hidden dangers. Even the green dye in the floral-patterned wallpapers of well-to-do homes and in the artificial leaves that adorned ladies' hats contained deadly arsenic. Everything was contaminated with toxic substances, from the food that was consumed each day to the very water that people drank. At the time Lister went off to UCL, London was drowning in its own filth.

In the midst of all this grime and muck, the city's citizens were trying to make improvements to their capital. Bloomsbury, the area surrounding the university where Lister would spend his time as a student, for example, had the pleasing aura of a freshly scrubbed baby. It was in a constant state of flux, growing at such a rapid pace that those who moved there in 1800 would hardly recognize it just a few decades later. When the young doctor Peter Mark Roget—who later became the author of the thesaurus that now bears his name—moved to 46 Great Russell Street at the turn of the century, he referred to the "pure" air and sprawling gardens surrounding his home. By the 1820s, the architect Robert Smirke had begun construction of the new British Museum on Roget's street. This imposing neoclassical structure would take twenty years to complete, during which time a cacophony of hammers, saws, and chisels rang out over Bloomsbury, shattering the neighborhood's formerly tranquil atmosphere that Roget had enjoyed so much.

The university was part of this urban growth. One balmy evening in early June 1825, the future lord chancellor of Great Britain Henry Brougham and several reforming members of Parliament sat down together at the Crown and Anchor Tavern in the Strand. There they conceived the project that was to become University College London (UCL). At this new institution, there were to be no religious stipulations. It was the first university in the country that didn't require its students to attend daily Anglican church services—a fact that suited Lister quite well. Later, rivals from King's College would label those who attended UCL "the Godless scum of Gower Street," referring to the thoroughfare on which the university was located.

The curriculum at UCL would be as radical as the secular foundations on which it was built, the founders decided. The university was to feature traditional subjects like those taught at Oxford and Cambridge, as well as new ones, such as geography, architecture, and modern history. The medical school, in particular, would have an advantage over the two other universities due to its proximity to the Northern London Hospital (later known as University College Hospital), built six years after UCL was founded.

There were many who balked at the idea of a university being established in London. The satirical newspaper *John Bull* questioned the suitability of the raucous city as a place in which to educate Britain's young minds. With trademark sarcasm, the newspaper quipped, "The morality of London, its quietude and salubrity, appear to combine to render the Capital the most convenient place for the education of youth." The article continued by imagining that the university would be built in the notorious slums near Westminster Abbey named Tothill Fields; "in order to meet any objections which heads of families may make to the perilous exposure of their sons to the casualties arising from crowded streets, a large body of plain respectable females, of the middle age, will be engaged to attend students to and from the College in the mornings and evenings of each day." Amid protests and concerns, however, the edifice of UCL was built, and the school began accepting students in October 1828.

—

THE UNIVERSITY WAS still in its infancy when Joseph Lister first arrived there in 1844. UCL had only three faculties: arts, medicine, and law. In keeping with his father's wishes, Lister completed an arts degree first, which was akin to a modern-day liberal arts foundation, consisting of a variety of courses in history, literature, mathematics, and science. This was an unconventional route into surgery because most students bypassed this step altogether in the 1840s and jumped right into a medical degree. Later in life, Lister would credit his broad background for his ability to connect scientific theories to medical practice.

At five feet ten inches, Lister was taller than most of his classmates. Those who knew him often commented on his striking stature and the gracefulness with which he moved. He was classically handsome at this age, with a straight nose, full lips, and brown wavy hair. He had a nervous energy about him that became more pronounced in the company of others. Hector Charles Cameron—one of Lister's biographers and a friend in later years—recalled the first time he met the future surgeon: "When I was admitted to the drawing-room Lister was standing with his back to the fire, tea cup in hand. As I remember him he was nearly always standing. . . . If for a few minutes he was seated, some new turn in the conversation seemed inevitably to force him to his feet."

Lister's mind was in a constant whirl of activity. When he was agitated or embarrassed, the corner of his mouth twitched, and a stammer that had plagued him in his early childhood would return. Despite this inner turbulence, Lister was described by the Stewart of Halifax as having an "indescribable air of gentleness, verging on shyness." A friend would later write of him, "He lived in the world of his thoughts, modest, unmasterful, unassuming."

Lister was a sober character, made all the more so by his upbringing. His community's religious teachings stipulated that people of his faith wear somber colors at all times, and address others using antiquated pronouns such as "thee" and "thou." As a child, Lister was surrounded by a sea of black coats and broad-brimmed hats, which the men of the family never removed, even during church services. The women dressed in plain garments with folded kerchiefs around

the neck and plain shawls on their shoulders. They wore white mus-
lin caps known as coal-scuttle bonnets. When Lister headed off to
university, he donned muted colors in deference to his faith, which,
among the more fashionable students of his class, no doubt made
him stand out as much as his height.

Shortly after arriving at UCL, Lister took up residence at
28 London Street, near the university, and lived there with a fellow
Quaker named Edward Palmer, who was eight years his senior. Palmer
was one of Robert Liston's assistants, in fact, and was described by
those who knew him as a "man in straightened [sic] circumstances
but with a real enthusiasm for the surgeon's profession." The two
quickly became friends. It was partly due to Palmer's influence that
Lister was able to attend Liston's historic experiment with ether on
December 21, 1846. That Lister was there at all suggests that this
was not his first time attending a medical lecture; it's unlikely that
the great Liston would have admitted him that afternoon had he not
already been acquainted with him. Indeed, Lister began his study of
anatomy several months *before* he finished his bachelor's in arts. In
his account books from the last quarter of that year, Lister notes
costs for the purchase of "forceps and sharpening knives," as well as
payment of eleven shillings, to a mysterious "U.L.," for a body part
that he dissected. His eagerness to begin his medical education was
apparent to all who knew him in his early years.

There was a darker side to Edward Palmer's personality that
didn't benefit Lister. In 1847, the two men moved to 2 Bedford Place
in Ampthill Square and were joined by John Hodgkin—nephew of
the famous Dr. Thomas Hodgkin, who was the first to describe the
very rare form of lymphoma that now bears his name. The Hodg-
kins and the Listers had long been friends, bonding over their shared
faith. The two boys had attended Grove House together, a boarding
school in Tottenham that taught a rather advanced curriculum for its

time, focusing not just on the classics but also on mathematics, natural science, and modern languages. Hodgkin, who was five years younger than Lister, called their rooms in Ampthill Square "dingy" and found his two housemates "far too mature and grave," which made "life a time of depression and joylessness." He was not as taken with Edward Palmer as his childhood friend seemed to be when Hodgkin first arrived at UCL. The young man referred to Palmer as a "curious being . . . peculiar . . . undoubtedly an odd man." Although Palmer was extremely devout, Hodgkin didn't think his oddity was especially connected with his religion. Most unsettling to Hodgkin was the fact that Lister became more withdrawn the longer he lived under Palmer's supervision. Aside from attending lectures, he seemed to take increasingly less interest in extracurricular activities, instead choosing to work hard in rather gloomy surroundings. And Palmer, who would become unhinged in later life and end his days in a mental institution, was hardly a cheerful influence in the aspiring surgeon's life. Hodgkin warned that he didn't think Palmer was "a very suitable companion even for Lister."

Both Lister and Palmer stood in contrast to many of their peers. In an address to incoming medical students, one of the surgical instructors at UCL warned about the "snares which notoriously lie in wait for the youthful traveler when he has left his parental hearth, and is wandering through the high-ways and by-ways—the broad streets and narrow alleys—of a great and over-peopled city." He railed against "vicious habits" like gambling, theatergoing, and drinking, declaring that they were "more contagious than leprosy of old, and disfigure the mind, more than that Eastern plague ever did the body." The instructor urged the incoming class to resist these vices and instead seek to uncover scientific truths through diligent study of anatomy, physiology, and chemistry.

His warnings were not misplaced.

At the time, the term "medical student" had become a "by-word for vulgar riot and dissipation," according to the physician William Augustus Guy. This sentiment was universal. An American journalist observed that medical students in New York were "apt to be lawless, exuberant, and addicted to nocturnal activities." They were often a rough-looking lot who congregated in cheap lodgings and inns surrounding the great teaching hospitals. They dressed fashionably—almost gaudily—except for their distinctly grimy shirts. They walked around with cigars hanging from their mouths: an indulgence, but one that was a necessity for masking the smell of decay that permeated their clothes after time spent in the dissection room. They were the brawling, boozing, boisterous types, judging by the number of warnings against bad behavior that instructors gave to their pupils.

Of course, not everyone at UCL was a raffish youngblood. Some, like Lister, were hardworking and diligent. They lived frugally, hocking watches in the local pawnbrokers' shops that dotted the narrow streets surrounding the university to pay for medical equipment. Others visited cutlers like J. H. Savigny, whose shop established in 1800 on the Strand was the first in London to specialize in surgical instruments. Places like this purported to sell scalpels, knives, and saws that, according to one British newspaper, were "wrought to such a degree of accuracy, as will greatly lessen the pain of the patient, and totally remove all apprehension of disappointment in the operator."

More than anything, what separated surgical students from the rest of the student body was the instruments they carried. Surgery was still a manual craft. It was a matter of technique, not technology. The instrument case of a newly qualified surgeon consisted of knives, bone saws, forceps, probes, hooks, needles, ligatures, and lancets, the latter being especially important given the persistent popularity of bloodletting in the Victorian period. Many surgeons also carried pocket cases of instruments with them, which they used for minor procedures, usually when making house calls.

The amputation knife assumed an almost mythical place in the surgeon's kit. It was one of the few instruments that underwent significant design changes in the first half of the nineteenth century. This was due in part to the changing nature of amputations. Older surgeons preferred the circular method, which involved making a sweeping incision around the circumference of the limb, pulling away the skin and muscle, and sawing through the bone. This called for a heavy knife with a curved, broad blade. Later generations, however, preferred what they called the flap method. Liston performed the flap method on the etherized Churchill in 1846. By the 1820s, the amputation knife was already thinner and lighter, with a straight blade reflecting the growing popularity of this technique. It involved "transfixing," which essentially required the surgeon to stab the patient, pushing the amputation knife downward into the limb before drawing it back upward and then piercing the skin from the underside of the incision.

Some surgeons customized their knives to suit their preferred techniques. Robert Liston—who was said to carry his scalpels up his coat sleeve to keep them warm—designed his very own amputation knife, which was considerably larger than the norm, with a blade fourteen inches long and one and a quarter inches wide. The dagger's point, the last two inches of which were razor-sharp, was created to cut through the skin, thick muscles, tendons, and tissues of the thigh with a single slice. It is little wonder that for Jack the Ripper, the "Liston knife" was the weapon of choice for the gutting of victims during his killing spree in 1888.

Instruments like the amputation knife of Lister's student days were havens for bacteria. Fashion often trumped function. Many had decorative etchings and were stored in velvet cases, which bore bloodstains from past operations. The surgeon William Fergusson recommended that the handles of surgical instruments be made of ebony, because this would be easier to grip when cutting through slippery bundles of veins and arteries. Traditional materials such as wood, ivory, and tortoiseshell also continued to be used in the nineteenth century, even after an upsurge in the production of metal instruments. As late as 1897, one catalogue stated, "We do not think that the day when metal-handled instruments will replace ebony and ivory is near at hand."

Lister's first instrument case had everything a novice surgeon would need at the start of his training: bone saws to hack off limbs; forceps to pick apart tissue; probes to root out bullets and foreign bodies. But there was one tool Lister had carried with him to UCL that very few in his class possessed: his microscope. Under his father's tutelage, he had grown into a very capable microscopist and learned to trust in the scientific instrument's powers.

Many of Lister's instructors still believed the microscope was not only superfluous to a study of surgery but also a threat to the medical establishment itself. Even with improvements like Joseph Jackson's achromatic lens, the instrument continued to be regarded with suspicion by those within the medical community, many of whom lacked the skill and training to operate one effectively. What revelations did the microscope offer? Surely all relevant signs and symptoms could be observed with the naked eye. And could any of these microscopic discoveries actually lead to the effective treatment of patients? Unless the instrument offered clear benefits that were applicable to the practice of medicine and surgery, most concluded that there was no reason to waste time with it.

Still, it was difficult for British doctors to deny the important advances made in pathology on the Continent due to the microscope. The French, in particular, were making discoveries at an extraordinary pace with the aid of the scientific instrument, owing partly to the rise of large hospitals in Paris during the French Revolution. By 1788, there were 20,341 patients residing in forty-eight different hospitals around the city: an unprecedented number unmatched anywhere else in the world. A large percentage of these people would succumb to their infirmities. Because they were often poor, their bodies went unclaimed and fell into the hands of anatomists like Marie François Xavier Bichat, who reportedly carved up no fewer than six hundred bodies in the winter of 1801–1802.

Bichat's research led him to conclude that the seat of disease was inside the body and that tissues were distinct entities that could be compromised. This was a departure from prevailing beliefs that disease attacked whole organs or the entire body. Remarkably, Bichat was able to describe and name twenty-one membranes in the human body, including connective, muscle, and nerve tissue, before he died accidentally in 1802 after falling down the steps of his own hospital.

In the early decades of the nineteenth century, French physicians began using the microscope more and more. The physician Pierre Rayer performed microscopic and chemical analyses of urine for the first time in history. The physiologist and pharmacologist François Magendie began using the instrument as a teaching tool in his physiology classes, and the physicians Gabriel Andral and Jules Gavarret started to analyze blood under the lens. By the time Lister was entering medical school, some Parisian physicians were even using microscopes to diagnose diseases of the skin, blood, kidneys, and urogenital system.

Back in England, the debate continued to rage over the advantages of microscopic pathological anatomy. Lister, however, was his father's son. At UCL, he showed himself to have a better grasp of the complex instrument's workings than most of his professors. Writing to his father about a lecture he attended on optical instruments, he remarked that the instructor "spoke of the improvements introduced by thee, and certainly gave thee the full credit for the whole revolution in microscopic excellence and observation, and said, moreover, that these improvements were the happiest instance of the application of experiment and observation to the construction of the Microscope; also, that thy experiments had been most skilfully executed."

And yet Lister wasn't entirely satisfied with the lecture. To his dismay, the instructor concluded damningly that students should remain skeptical about the microscope's useful application in medicine, because the results of any experiments with it were likely to be flawed as long as improvements were still needed. A querulous Lister complained to his father that the lecture was "rather a disappointment to me, and I fancy to others too."

But Lister would not be easily deterred. He turned his attention to the microscopic structure of muscle after obtaining a fresh portion of human iris from UCL's professor Wharton Jones. He noted pigment granules in the lens as well as in the iris. Later, he turned his attention to the muscular tissue within hair follicles and devised a new method for making vertical sections thin enough to be observed satisfactorily under the microscope: "By compressing a portion [of the scalp] between two thin pieces of deal [wood], and cutting off with a sharp razor fine shavings of wood and scalp together, moderately thin sections may be obtained." From these experiments, Lister eventually published two papers in the *Quarterly Journal of Microscopical Science*. These were the first of many investigations he would conduct with the microscope during his surgical career.

Years later, Lister's supervisor had little to say about his subordinate, remarking that he was "too shy and reserved to be more than an acquaintance" when the two were working alongside each other at

University College Hospital in 1851. That said, his supervisor did recall something that distinguished Lister from the other students: "He had a better microscope than any man in college." It was this very instrument that would eventually help him unlock the medical mystery that had been plaguing his profession for centuries.

2.

HOUSES OF DEATH

What a charming task, to sit quietly down in the apartment and take apart this master-piece of workmanship; to call each piece by its proper name; know its proper place and work; to wonder over the multitude of organs pressed together, so diverse in operations, yet each executing its appointed task in the grand confederation.

—D. HAYES AGNEW

A HALO OF LIGHT from a gas lamp illuminated the corpse lying on the table at the back of the room. The body had already been mutilated beyond recognition, its abdomen hacked away by the knives of eager students who afterward carelessly tossed the decomposing organs back into the gory cavity. The top of the cadaver's skull had been removed and was now sitting on a stool next to its deceased owner. The brain had begun to degrade into a gray paste days before.

Early in Lister's medical studies, he came face-to-face with a similar scene at UCL. A central walkway split the dingy dissection room in half, with five wooden tables on either side. Cadavers were left with their incised heads hanging over the edges, which caused blood to gather in congealed puddles below. A thick layer of sawdust covered the floor, making the deadhouse disconcertingly quiet to those who entered it. "Not a sound could be heard even of my own feet. . . . There was only that dull and rolling sound of the traffic in the streets which is peculiar to London, and which came dismally down through the ventilators in the roof," a fellow student observed.

Although UCL and its hospital were still relatively new in 1847, its dissection room was just as grim as those found in older institutions. It harbored all kinds of horrible sights, sounds, and smells. When Lister sliced into the abdomen of a cadaver—its recesses turgid with a thick soup of undigested food and fecal matter—he released a powerful mixture of fetid smells that would cleave to the inside of the nostrils for a considerable time after one had quit the scene. To make matters worse, there was an open fireplace at the end of the room, making it unbearably stuffy during the winter months when anatomy lessons commenced.

Unlike today, students could not escape the dead during their studies and often lived side by side with the bodies they dissected. Even those who did not live immediately adjacent to an anatomy school carried with them reminders of their gruesome activities, because neither gloves nor other forms of protective gear were worn inside the dissection room. Indeed, it was not uncommon to see a medical student with shreds of flesh, gut, or brains stuck to his clothing after his lessons were over.

The cadaver tested the courage and composure of anyone who dared set foot inside the deadhouse. Even the most seasoned dissectors could find themselves in pulse-quickening situations from time to time. The gynecological surgeon James Marion Sims recalled a terrifying incident from his student days. His instructor was performing a dissection by candlelight one evening when he accidentally knocked loose a chain that was wrapped around the corpse and anchored to the ceiling above the upper end of the table. The cadaver, pulled by the weight of its own lower limbs, "jerked to the floor in the upright posture" with its "arms forcibly thrown over" the dissector's shoulders. Just then, the candle, which had been resting on the dead man's chest, sputtered out, leaving the room in total darkness. Sims was astounded when his instructor calmly took hold of the body under its arms and placed it back on the table, before remarking that if it had been up to him, he'd have left the dead man to the force of gravity.

For the uninitiated, the dissection room was a waking nightmare. The French composer and former medical student Hector Berlioz jumped out of a window and ran home, later recalling that it was "as though Death himself and all his grisly band were hot on my heels" the first time he stepped into a dissection room. He described an overwhelming feeling of revulsion at the sight of "the limbs scattered about, the heads smirking, the skulls gaping, the bloody cesspool underfoot," and "the repulsive stench of the place." One of the worst sights, he thought, was of the rats nibbling on bleeding vertebrae and the swarms of sparrows pecking at the leftover scraps of spongy lung tissue. The profession was not for everyone.

But for those wishing to continue with their degrees, there was no avoiding the dissection room. Far from viewing it as repulsive, most students ultimately embraced the opportunity to carve up the dead when the time came to commence their anatomical lessons, and Lister was no exception. Theirs was a centuries-old battle between reason and superstition: a chance to shed light where there was still scientific darkness. Within the medical profession, the anatomist was often hailed as an explorer boldly traveling into regions that had been largely unknown to the scientific world only half a century earlier. One contemporary wrote that through dissection, the anatomist "forced the dead human body to disclose its secrets for the benefit of the living." It was a rite of passage through which one gained membership in the medical fraternity.

Little by little, students began to view the bodies set before them not as people but as objects. This ability to divorce oneself emotionally came to characterize the mind-set of the medical community. In *The Pickwick Papers*, Charles Dickens describes a fictional but entirely credible conversation between two medical students on a frosty Christmas morning. "Have you finished that leg yet?" asks Benjamin Allen. "Nearly," replies his colleague Bob Sawyer, "it's a very muscular one for a child's. . . . Nothing like dissecting to give one an appetite."

Today, we disparagingly call this apparent coldness clinical detachment, but in Lister's day it was described as a necessary inhumanity. The French anatomist Joseph-Guichard Duverney remarked that by "seeing and practicing" on dead bodies, "we lose foolish tenderness, so we can hear them cry, without any disorder." This was not simply a by-product of medical education. It was the goal.

As medical students became desensitized, they also became irreverent—much to the public's horror. Pranks in the deadhouse were so common that by the time Lister entered medical school, they had become a mark of the profession. *Harper's New Monthly Magazine* condemned the jet-black humor and indifference toward the dead that pervaded the dissection room. Some students completely overstepped the bounds of decency and used the rotting body parts of their allotted cadavers as weapons, fighting mock duels with the severed legs and arms. Others smuggled entrails out of the room and secreted them in places where they would shock and horrify the uninitiated when discovered. One surgeon remembered curious spectators visiting the dissection room when he was a student. These outsiders wore double-breasted jackets and often received in their tail pockets free donations of available appendages.

It wasn't all frivolity. Cutting open dead bodies also carried with it many physical risks, some of which were fatal. William Tennant Gairdner, a professor at the University of Glasgow, addressed an incoming class with this dire message: "Not a single session has passed over our heads since I was appointed to my office among you, that has not paid its tax of life to the great Reaper, whose harvest is always ready, whose sickle is never weary."

Jacob Bigelow—professor of surgery at Harvard University and father of Henry Jacob Bigelow, who later witnessed William T. G. Morton's operation with ether—also warned future medical students about the poisonous effects of a slight wound or crack in the skin made by the dissecting knife. These so-called pinprick cuts were a fast way to an early grave. The dangers were always present, even for the most experienced anatomists. Death was often inescapable for those trying their hardest to prevent it.

The living, in the form of diseased patients, were also taking a toll on those on the front line of medicine. Mortality rates among medical students and young doctors were high. Between 1843 and 1859, forty-one young men died after contracting fatal infections at St. Bartholomew's Hospital, before ever qualifying as doctors. Those who succumbed in this manner were often eulogized as martyrs who had made the ultimate sacrifice in order to advance anatomical knowledge. Even those who survived often suffered some sort of illness during their hospital residencies. Indeed, the challenges were so great for those entering the profession that the surgeon John Abernethy frequently concluded his lectures by uttering bleakly, "God help you all. What will become of you?"

. . .

It wasn't long before Lister experienced the physical dangers of his occupation. He was ensconced in his medical studies when he noticed tiny white pustules on the backs of his hands. It could only be one thing: smallpox.

He was all too familiar with the telltale signs of this terrible disease because his brother John had contracted smallpox a few years earlier. Around a third of those who caught it died. Those who survived were often left with disfiguring scars. One contemporary wrote that the "hideous traces of its power" haunted its victims, "turning the babe into a changeling at which the mother shuddered, and making the eyes and cheeks of the betrothed maiden objects of horror to the lover." For this reason, smallpox was one of the most feared diseases of the nineteenth century.

John survived but developed an unrelated brain tumor shortly afterward. He suffered for several years—first losing his eyesight, then the function of his legs—before finally dying in 1846 at the age of twenty-three. The death was especially hard on Lister's father, Joseph Jackson, who lost all enthusiasm for his work with the microscope as a result. He was never to return to it again. For Lister, it was the first time he had witnessed the true limitations of his profession, for there wasn't a doctor in the world who could operate successfully on John's brain tumor in the 1840s.

Despite the sheer terror accompanying the onset of smallpox, Lister's own case turned out to be mild, like his brother's. He recovered within a short period and didn't suffer any scarring on his face or hands. But his brush with death unnerved him and left dozens of questions about his own fate twisting in his mind. He turned more fervently to religion. His friend and fellow lodger John Hodgkin later wrote that Lister was passing through some religious conflict of the soul following his recovery from smallpox. His attention began to drift away from his studies at the university as he began to wonder whether his true vocation lay not with surgery but with the Quaker ministry. As a preacher, he could make a real difference. Medicine had done nothing to save his brother's life. Maybe the Quakers had been right to place greater trust in the healing power of nature than in the medical profession.

Lister's crisis of conscience reached its tipping point one Wednesday evening in 1847, when he and Hodgkin attended a Quaker gathering at the Friends Meeting House, located on Gracechurch Street, not far from campus. Hodgkin watched in astonishment as his friend stood up in the silent prayer meeting and said: "I will be with thee & keep thee: fear thou not." The only Quakers permitted to speak at meetings were ministers. By quoting passages from the Bible, Lister was indicating to those in his community (including Hodgkin) that he felt his destiny lay not in the operating theater—surrounded by blood and guts—but in the pulpit. Joseph Jackson immediately interceded. He didn't believe his son's otherwise laudable desire to do the Lord's work would be best served within the limits of the Quaker ministry. Instead, he urged Lister to continue with his medical studies and please God by helping the sick.

Yet Lister slipped deeper and deeper into depression. Unable to function, he left UCL abruptly in March 1848. His mental collapse was a manifestation of the depression that would dog him his entire life. One of his contemporaries later said of him that a "cloud of seriousness" always hung over Lister and "tempered all he did." He carried with him a "garment of sadness which he seemed seldom to discard," brought on by his own overwhelming "sense of responsibility that lay like a burden upon his soul."

While it may seem anachronistic, the term "nervous breakdown" was used by Lister's nephew and biographer Rickman John Godlee later to describe this period of his uncle's life. Throughout Victoria's reign, most medical practitioners treated nervous disorders by administering concoctions containing dangerous ingredients, including morphine, strychnine, quinine, codeine, atropine, mercury, and even arsenic, which was added to the London *Pharmacopoeia* in 1809. The use of these nerve tonics, as they were called, was advocated by adherents of the prevalent medical orthodoxy of the time known as allopathy, meaning "other than the disease." In short, the theory held that the best way to treat a disease was to produce the somatic condition opposite to the pathological state in question. With a fever, for instance, one had to cool the body down. With disorders of the mind, one had to restore strength and firmness to the patient's frayed nerves.

"Naturopathy"—the treatment of disease through the promotion of the body's own healing powers—also played a significant role in Victorian medicine. Doctors put great stock in a change of air and scenery to combat what they considered the source of shattered nerves: stress, overwork, and mental anxiety. It was important that patients remove themselves from the environment in which they had broken down.

This was the path Lister chose. In late April, Lister traveled with Hodgkin to the Isle of Wight on England's south coast, where they paid a visit to the old Needles Lighthouse, perched on a cliff 472 feet above Scratchell's Bay. By June, he had arrived in Ilfracombe, a beautiful village in Somerset on the shoreline of the Bristol Channel. From there, he accepted an invitation to visit Ireland from a prosperous merchant, Thomas Pim. The Pims were prominent Quakers in Monkstown, which was near Dublin and something of a stronghold for the Society of Friends in that part of Ireland. Joseph Jackson wrote to his son that he hoped these excursions were helping to restore Lister's mental state: "The things that sometimes distress thee are really only the results of illness, following too close study . . . thy proper part now is to cherish a pious cheerful spirit, open to see & to enjoy the bounties and the beauties spread around us:—not to give way to turning thy thoughts upon thyself nor even at present to dwell long on serious things."

Lister traveled around Britain and Europe for twelve months before finally returning to London. In 1849, he overcame his inner demons and reenrolled at UCL, where a passion for surgery was reborn in him. Lister began pursuing his anatomical studies outside the dissection room in his spare time, acquiring various body parts from bone collectors and medical suppliers to further his understanding of human anatomy. These included a bladder, a thorax, and a head with partial spinal cord attached, which he bought for twelve shillings and sixpence. In December of that year, he purchased a complete human skeleton from his former roommate Edward Palmer for five pounds, which he paid off over the next two years.

After the first year of medical school, Lister began his residency at University College Hospital in October 1850. Several months later, the medical committee offered him the position of surgical dresser to John Eric Erichsen, the hospital's senior surgeon. Lister accepted, despite having turned the post down earlier on account of his poor health.

The best that can be said about Victorian hospitals is that they were a *slight* improvement over their Georgian predecessors. That's hardly a ringing endorsement when one considers that a hospital's "Chief Bug-Catcher"—whose job it was to rid the mattresses of lice—was paid more than its surgeons.

Admittedly, a number of London hospitals in the first half of the nineteenth century were rebuilt or extended in line with the demands placed upon them by the city's growing population. For instance, St. Thomas' Hospital received a new anatomical theater and museum in 1813; and St. Bartholomew's Hospital underwent several structural improvements between 1822 and 1854, which increased the number of patients it could receive. Three teaching hospitals were also built during this time, including University College Hospital in 1834.

Despite these changes—or because these enlargements suddenly brought hundreds of patients into proximity with one another—hospitals were known by the public as "Houses of Death." Some only admitted patients who brought with them money to cover their almost inevitable burial. Others, like St. Thomas', charged double if the person in question was deemed "foul" by the admissions officer. The surgeon James Y. Simpson remarked as late as 1869 that a "soldier has more chance of survival on the field of Waterloo than a man who goes into hospital."

In spite of token efforts to make hospitals cleaner, most remained overcrowded, grimy, and poorly managed. They were breeding grounds for infection and provided only the most primitive facilities for the sick and the dying, many of whom were housed on wards with little ventilation or access to clean water. Surgical incisions made in large city hospitals were so vulnerable to infection that operations were restricted to only the most urgent cases. The sick often languished in filth for long periods before they received medical attention, because most hospitals were disastrously understaffed. In 1825, visitors to St. George's Hospital discovered mushrooms and maggots thriving in the damp, dirty sheets of a patient recovering from a compound fracture. The afflicted man, believing this to be the norm, had not complained about the conditions, nor had any of his fellow ward mates thought the squalor especially noteworthy.

Worst of all was the fact that hospitals constantly reeked of piss, shit, and vomit. A sickening odor permeated every surgical ward. The smell was so offensive that doctors sometimes walked around with handkerchiefs pressed to their noses. It was this affront to the senses that most tested surgical students on their first day in the hospital.

Berkeley Moynihan—one of the first surgeons in England to use rubber gloves—recalled how he and his colleagues used to throw off their own jackets when entering the operating theater and don an ancient frock that was often stiff with dried blood and pus. It had belonged to a retired member of staff and was worn as a badge of honor by his proud successors, as were many items of surgical clothing.

Pregnant women who suffered vaginal tears during delivery were especially at risk in these dangerous environments because these wounds provided welcome openings for the bacteria that doctors and surgeons carried on them wherever they went. In England and Wales in the 1840s, approximately 3,000 mothers died each year from bacterial infections such as puerperal fever (also known as childbed fever). This amounted to roughly 1 death for every 210 confinements. Many women also died from pelvic abscesses, hemorrhaging, or peritonitis—the latter being a terrible condition in which bacteria travel through the bloodstream and inflame the peritoneum, the lining of the abdomen.

Because surgeons saw suffering on a daily basis, very few felt any need to address an issue that they saw as inevitable and commonplace. Most surgeons were interested in the individual bodies of their patients, not hospital populations and statistics. They were largely unconcerned with the causes of diseases, choosing instead to focus on diagnosis, prognosis, and treatment. Lister, however, would soon form his own opinions about the parlous state of hospital wards and about what could be done to address what he saw as a growing humanitarian crisis.

Many of the surgeons with whom Lister came into contact in those early years as a medical student were fatalistic about their ability to help patients and improve hospitals. John Eric Erichsen—the senior surgeon at University College Hospital—was one such practitioner.

Erichsen was a lean man with dark hair and prominent examples of the era's trademark whiskers. He had limpid, inquisitive eyes set in a kindly face, with a sloping forehead, a long nose, and a slight turn to the lips. Unlike many of his colleagues, he was not a very skilled operator. Rather, he built his reputation on his writing and on his teaching. His most successful book, *The Science and Art of Surgery*, ran into nine editions and was the leading textbook on the subject for several decades. It was translated into German, Italian, and Spanish and held in such high regard in America that a copy of it was given to every medical officer in the federal army during the Civil War.

But Erichsen was shortsighted about the future of surgery, which he believed was rapidly approaching the limits of its powers by the middle of the nineteenth century. History will remember the whiskered surgeon for his misguided prediction: "There cannot always be fresh fields of conquest by the knife; there must be portions of the human frame that will ever remain sacred from its intrusions, at least in the surgeon's hands. That we have already, if not quite, reached these final limits, there can be little question. The abdomen, the chest, and the brain will be forever shut from the intrusion of the wise and humane surgeon."

Wayward prophecies aside, Erichsen did recognize the momentous transformation that the surgeon was currently undergoing as a result of recent educational reforms. Whereas before the surgeon was a glorified butcher with steady hands, now he was a skilled operator, guided by greater knowledge. Erichsen observed, "It is long since the *hand* has been [the surgeon's] sole dependence; and it is now by the *head*, as much or more than by the hand, that he exercises his avocation."

Erichsen had come by his position via the kind of misfortune that exemplified the perils of his profession. Four years earlier, his predecessor John Phillips Potter had entered the dissection room to anatomize the body of the circus performer and dwarf Harvey Leach, known by many in London as the "Gnome Fly" due to his propensity to flit around the stage like a winged insect.

Leach, who was often billed as the "shortest man in the world," had made a name for himself as a performing oddity. In addition to his small stature, one of his legs was eighteen inches long while the other measured twenty-four inches, and when he walked, his arms brushed against the ground like an ape's. According to one of his contemporaries, Leach appeared "like a head and trunk, moving about on castors."

Leach's strange appearance eventually attracted the attention of the American showman and hoaxer P. T. Barnum, founder of the Barnum & Bailey Circus. Barnum dressed the dwarf in the skin of a wild beast and covered the walls of London with placards that read "What Is It?" Unbeknownst to Barnum, Leach was so recognizable at that point in his career that people guessed the true identity of this mysterious "beast" within days. Despite this initial bungle, Barnum retained Leach as a performer, until the forty-six-year-old man died as the result of an injured hip that had become infected. At a time when people went to great lengths to ensure their bodies remained intact after death, Leach allegedly stipulated that his be handed over to those who were most likely to cut him up. According to an Australian newspaper, Leach requested that his corpse "be presented to Dr. Liston, the eminent surgeon, not to be buried, but embalmed and kept in a glass case, as the doctor had been a particular friend to him." Another newspaper in Britain said that Leach had "bequeathed his body over to his most intimate friend and companion, Mr. Potter," which seems more likely given the fact that it was Potter who ultimately performed the dissection. Whatever the circumstances under which his body was obtained, and whatever his actual wishes might have been, an anatomization of Leach went ahead on April 22, 1847.

Potter, who had proven himself to be a lively, brilliant, and excellent teacher, had just that week been appointed assistant surgeon at University College Hospital. It was said that his kindness and zeal in his previous role as demonstrator of anatomy had made him popular with faculty and students alike, and Lister was among his admirers. As Potter cut into Leach's stiff body, he noted: "It seems as though the thigh-bones and muscles had disappeared, and the knee-joints been raised up to the hips." According to Potter, in place of a normal structure, Leach appeared to have "an immensely strong bone of triangular form, with the base upwards, . . . knit to the hip with very strong ligaments." Potter reckoned it was because of this that the famous circus performer could jump ten feet into the air.

Potter carefully sliced his way deeper into the corpse, pausing to make meticulous notes as he did so. Suddenly his lancet slipped, causing him to puncture the knuckle of his forefinger. Unaware of the precarious situation he now found himself in, Potter continued with the anatomization. Days later, the young surgeon began to develop pyemia, a form of septicemia that results in the development of widespread abscesses all over the body—a condition doubtless brought on by his exposure to Leach's bacteria-riddled corpse. The infection traveled up his arm, eventually spreading all over his body. Over the next three weeks, five doctors—including Robert Liston—attended Potter's bedside, purportedly draining three pints of pus from his sacral region and an additional two pints from his chest, before the young man finally died. The official report concluded that had Potter eaten breakfast before rushing into the dissection room, he might have lived, because a full stomach would have aided the absorption of the toxic substances that had entered his body when dissecting Leach. In an era that knew nothing of germs, this explanation seemed entirely plausible.

Two hundred mourners followed Potter's coffin into the sprawling expanse of London's Kensal Green Cemetery for his funeral, turning out to pay their respects to the man who had shown so much promise in his short career. *The Lancet* later lamented that it was "a most melancholy and disheartening instance of brilliant talent and promise blighted in the blood." Potter's misfortune, however, was Erichsen's good luck. The dirt shoveled back into poor Potter's grave had barely settled before the Danish-born surgeon stepped into his dead colleague's shoes.

As it turned out, 1847 was a bad year for many of the hospital's surgeons. On December 7—nearly one year after his historic operation with ether—the great surgeon Robert Liston died unexpectedly of an aortic aneurysm at the age of fifty-three. His death was felt deeply by the medical staff at University College Hospital, many of whom resigned their positions in search of other surgical giants to follow. The loss of such well-loved instructors as Potter and Liston also diminished the number of students wishing to study there, which in turn led to a substantial decrease in revenue. By the end of the 1840s, the hospital was three thousand pounds in debt and had to scale back the number of beds from 130 to 100. Only half of these were designated for surgical cases.

Erichsen was quickly promoted. His appointment to the chair of surgery in 1850 at the age of thirty-two so offended his senior colleague Richard Quain that the latter refused to talk to Erichsen for fifteen years. Such is the timelessness of hospital politics. Erichsen had three dressers assigned to him when Lister came on board as a fourth. The dressers were required to take a case history for each patient, prepare diet tables, and assist in postmortem examinations. Lister and his three colleagues reported to Erichsen's house surgeon, an eccentric young man named Henry Thompson who later became known in London for hosting "octaves"—dinners of eight courses for eight people served at eight o'clock. Thompson supervised the dressers and attended to Erichsen's patients each morning. As a fully qualified surgeon, he also assisted Erichsen with operations, whereas Lister and the other dressers could not.

All five men lived in the housing quarters within the hospital. It was a healthy change from the stifling existence Lister had known as a lodger in Edward Palmer's house while studying for his arts degree. For the first time in his life, Lister came into contact with young men from differing educational and religious backgrounds who held many views that were at odds with his own. He thrived in this new environment and became an active member of the student body. Partly in an attempt to rid himself of the stammer that had preceded his breakdown, Lister joined the Medical Society, where he engaged in lively debates with other students over the merits of the microscope as a tool for medical research. He also led a scathing attack on homeopathic medicine, which he argued was "perfectly untenable scientifically." Such was his oratorial heft that a year after he joined, he was elected president of the society.

Back at the hospital, Lister had only been acting as Erichsen's dresser for a short period when there was an outbreak of erysipelas, an acute skin infection sometimes referred to as "St. Anthony's Fire" because it turns the skin bright red and shiny. The condition is caused by the streptococcus bacterium and can develop rapidly over a period of a few hours, causing high fevers, tremors, and eventually death. Most surgeons at this time considered erysipelas all but incurable. Its terrible effects were ubiquitous. It was so contagious that institutions like Blockley Almshouse in Philadelphia (later Philadelphia General Hospital) imposed a moratorium on operations from January until March, when they believed erysipelas was at its seasonal peak.

Lister was more familiar with the condition than most of his classmates. His mother, Isabella, had suffered from recurring outbreaks of erysipelas since Lister was a small boy. (It was probably due to her ongoing ill health that Lister himself became something of a hypochondriac later in life. The most obvious outward manifestation of his neurosis was a fixation with his shoes, which he always ensured had unusually thick soles. One of his friends speculated this was a result of Lister's "unreasoned dread of wet feet," which most people of his generation believed were the root of sickness.)

Erysipelas was one of four major infections that plagued hospitals in the nineteenth century. The other three were hospital gangrene (ulcers that lead to decay of flesh, muscle, and bone), septicemia (blood poisoning), and pyemia (development of pus-filled abscesses). Any one of these conditions could prove fatal depending on a wide range of factors, not least the age and general health of the sufferer. The increase in infection and suppuration brought on by "the big four" later became known as hospitalism, which the medical community increasingly blamed on the establishment of large urban hospitals wherein patients found themselves in close contact with one another. Although the construction of these buildings met the needs of a rapidly growing population, many doctors believed that hospitals counteracted surgical advancements, because a majority of patients died of infections they would not otherwise have contracted had they not been admitted in the first place. Indeed, one contemporary argued that the medical community could not hope for "progress in the public practice of the healing art, till our system of hospitalism is more or less changed and revolutionized."

The problem was that no one knew exactly how infectious diseases were transmitted. By the 1840s, the formulation of an effectual public health policy was hostage to a debate between the so-called contagionists and anti-contagionists. The former posited that disease was communicated from person to person or via the medium of goods being shipped in from pestilent areas of the world. Contagionists were vague about the agent by which disease was passed. Some suggested it was a chemical or even small "invisible bullets." Others thought it might be transmitted via an "animalcule," a catchall term for small organisms. Contagionists maintained that the only way to prevent and control epidemic diseases was through the use of quarantines and trade restrictions. Contagionism seemed plausible when it came to diseases such as smallpox, where fluid in the pustules could easily be seen as the mode of transmission; however, it did little to explain sicknesses that arose through indirect contact, like cholera or yellow fever.

On the other side were the anti-contagionists, who believed disease was generated spontaneously from filth and decaying matter, in a process known as pythogenesis, and then transmitted through the air via poisonous vapors, or miasma. (That the name of a disease like malaria derives from the Italian words *mala*, or "bad," and *aria*, or "air," suggests that people believed the disease had miasmic origins.) Anti-contagionism was popular among the medical elite, who opposed the draconian restrictions on free trade that contagionists advocated during epidemics. Proponents of anti-contagionism believed their theory was grounded in sound observation. One only had to look to the squalid conditions of an overcrowded city to recognize that highly populated areas were most often at the epicenter of outbreaks. In 1844, the physician Neil Arnott summarized anti-contagionism when he argued that the immediate and chief cause of disease in metropolitan areas was "the poison of atmospheric impurity arising from the accumulation in and around [people's] dwellings of the decomposing remnants of the substances used for food and from the impurities given out from their own bodies." Anti-contagionists advocated their own program of prevention and control that placed an emphasis on environmental improvements that would eradicate the conditions in which diseases could arise.

While many medical practitioners recognized that neither of the two theories provided a comprehensive explanation for how infectious diseases spread, most hospital surgeons sided with the anti-contagionists by pointing to contaminated air in overcrowded wards as the cause of hospitalism. The French called the phenomenon *l'intoxication nosocomiale* (hospital poisoning). At University College Hospital, Erichsen concurred. He maintained that patients were infected by miasma arising from corrupt wounds. The air, he thought, would become saturated with poisonous gases, which in turn were inhaled by patients: this miasma might appear "at any season of the year, and under any circumstances, acquire extreme virulence, if the crowding together of the operated or injured . . . be excessive." Erichsen estimated that more than seven patients with an infected wound in a fourteen-bed ward could lead to an irreversible outbreak of any one of the four principal hospital diseases. He could hardly be blamed for thinking so.

While comparing mortality rates of country practitioners with those operating in the large, urban hospitals of London and Edinburgh during this period, the obstetrician James Y. Simpson discovered some shocking differences. Of twenty-three double amputations performed on patients in the countryside over a twelve-month period, only seven died. Although this statistic may seem high, it is low when compared with the mortality rate at the Royal Infirmary of Edinburgh for the same period. Of the eleven patients who received double amputations there during this time, a shocking ten of these died. A further breakdown shows that the leading cause of death in amputees in the countryside during the mid-nineteenth century was shock and exhaustion, whereas the leading cause of death in the urban hospitals was postoperative infection. Many surgeons began to question the impact that large hospitals were having on their patients' ability to recover.

University College Hospital had a swift isolation policy when it came to dealing with hospitalism's conditions. *The Lancet* reported that the hospital "had been extremely healthy, and quite free from any erysipelas originating within its walls," when Lister came to work for Erichsen in January 1851. And yet it was during that same month that a patient presenting with necrosis of the legs was brought into the wards from the Islington workhouse. He also happened to be infected with erysipelas. Although he only occupied the bed for two hours before Erichsen ordered his isolation, it was too late. The damage was done. Within hours, the infection spread over the entire ward, killing numerous patients. The outbreak was finally contained when the infected patients were moved off the ward to a different area of the hospital.

Many of these victims would have undoubtedly been carried to the dissection room to be anatomized, emphasizing for Lister and his colleagues the apparently unbreakable nature of the cycle of disease and death, with the hospital ward forming its axis. Success or failure of treatment at a House of Death was a lottery. But occasionally, opportunities would arise for the surgeon to take the initiative to save lives in unexpected ways, as Lister would soon discover.

3.

THE SUTURED GUT

—

We should ask ourselves, whether, placed under similar circumstances, we should choose to submit to the pain and danger we are about to inflict.

—SIR ASTLEY COOPER

THE FLAME OF LISTER'S CANDLE flickered in the window of the casualty and outpatient department of University College Hospital at one o'clock on the morning of June 27, 1851. Other wards had recently installed gaslit ceiling pendants, but this area of the hospital still relied on candlelight. Candles had always been problematic in a medical setting. They provided inconsistent lighting, and surgeons were forced to bring them dangerously close to patients in order to inspect them properly. One of Erichsen's patients had only recently complained after hot wax dripped onto his neck during an examination.

Lister often took advantage of the quiet nocturnal hours to write up case notes and check on patients. On this particular night, however, there would be no peace. Suddenly, a commotion erupted on the street outside the hospital. Lister snatched the candle from the window, its light receding deeper into the building as his footsteps echoed on hardwood floors. The flame briefly illuminated each room he passed through as he strode toward the main entrance. Just then, the doors burst open. Lister raised the candle to reveal the face of a frantic policeman. In the officer's arms was an unconscious woman. She had been stabbed in the gut, and although the wound was small, slick coils of her intestines had started to protrude from her body. Lister was not just the most senior surgeon on duty. He was the *only* surgeon on duty.

He set the candle down and got to work.

The young woman now in Lister's care was Julia Sullivan, a mother of eight, who had fallen victim to her husband's alcohol-fueled temper. Domestic abuse was not a rarity in Victorian England. Wife-beating was a national pastime, and women like Julia were often treated like property by their husbands.

Some men even put their own wives and children up for sale after they tired of them. One deed for such a sale declared that a Mr. Osborn "does agree to part with my wife Mary Osborn and child to Mr William Sergeant for the sum of one pound, consideration of giving up all claim." In another instance, a journalist wrote of a butcher who had dragged his wife to Smithfield Market "with a halter about her neck, and one about her waist, which tied her to a railing." The husband ended up selling his wife to a "happy purchaser" who paid the man three guineas and a crown for "his departed rib." Between 1800 and 1850, there were more than two hundred recorded cases of wife sales in England. Undoubtedly, there were more that went unreported.

There was little legal protection for a victimized woman in the mid-nineteenth century. The editor of *The Times* criticized the lenient sentences handed out by magistrates of the court to abusive husbands, opining that the "conjugal tie appears to be considered as conferring on the man a certain degree of impunity for brutality towards the woman." These violent men lived in a society that turned a blind eye to their abuse. The general populace had grown so accustomed to the idea that men were allowed to beat women and children that it practically sanctioned this behavior. On May 31, 1850, a writer for *The Morning Chronicle* commented,

> It is evident to all who take any pains to read the indications
> of the feelings of the populace that they are impressed with
> the belief of their having a *right* to inflict almost any amount
> of corporal violence on *their* wife or *their* children. That
> anyone should claim to interfere with this supposed right
> causes them unaffected surprise. It is not *their* wife or child?
> Are they not entitled to do as they will with their own?
> These phrases are not, to their apprehension, metaphorical.
> The shoes on their feet, the cudgel in their hand, the horse
> or ass that carries their burden, the wife and children, all
> are "theirs" and all in the same sense.

This was the world in which Julia Sullivan lived when her fifty-nine-year-old husband, Jeremiah, lunged at her with a long, narrow-bladed knife that he had concealed in his sleeve, just an hour before she was rushed to University College Hospital.

The tension between the unhappy couple had been mounting for some time before the attack. Sullivan's alcoholism and violent outbursts had driven his wife from their home five weeks earlier. Flight was one of the few options available to Julia in 1851, when a woman's initiation of divorce proceedings was contingent on the husband's committing both adultery *and* assault (the same was not true for the husband). This could only be achieved by an Act of Parliament. And even if these criteria could be met, the expense of divorce was beyond the means of most lower-class women, who often lacked the funds to support themselves and risked being denied contact with their children should they obtain a legal separation. In Julia's case, being beaten on a regular basis by her alcoholic husband was simply not enough to warrant filing for divorce under English law.

Julia had recently moved out of her home and was sharing a room with an elderly widow in Camden Town, an area of London with a mixed crowd of poor working-class folk. Three weeks before the attack, a mob of local people had heard Sullivan shout obscenities and make threats against his wife's life on the new street where she lived. His behavior was paranoid and delusional, and he thought that Julia was having an affair. One man, a Francis Poltock, confronted Sullivan, telling him to go away and that his wife wouldn't come out and see him. According to court documents, Sullivan was seething with anger when he spat back, "If she don't let me come in I will *do* for her."

That night, Sullivan surprised Julia outside her apartment as she was coming home from work. He grabbed her and demanded she return home with him, before tapping his sleeve in a threatening manner. Julia, thinking this was strange, asked him what he had hidden in there. He sneered, "Why, you foolish woman, do you think I have anything in my jacket-sleeve to take away your life, and send my soul to the devil?"

The two fell into a blazing argument that brought the neighbor Bridget Bryan to the door to complain about the noise. Sullivan implored his wife to accompany him to a local pub. She refused, so he put his hand on her back and pushed her into the street. Bridget urged Julia to comply with Sullivan's wishes for the sake of peace, and all three walked to the pub. While there, the spouses resumed their fight after Julia once again refused to leave with Sullivan. At last, the two women left on their own and started to make their way back home. Just when they dared hope they were free of Sullivan and his drunken ranting, he leaped at them out of the shadows. Julia, who thought her husband was about to strike her, put her hands up to cover her face. It was then that he sank the knife deep into her belly, crying, "There, I have done that for you!"

As Julia lurched forward in pain, Bridget frantically put her hands underneath her friend's clothes to feel for the wound. She shouted, "Sullivan, you have killed your wife!" He stood there watching the scene unfold before replying, darkly, "Oh no, she is not dead yet."

Thomas Gentle, a police officer on duty that night, later recalled seeing Julia limping down the street, escorted by Sullivan and her neighbor. When he asked her what was wrong, she groaned, "Oh, policeman, my life is in your hands; this man has stabbed me," indicating her husband standing next to her. Instinctively, she put her hand on her abdomen. It was then that she made a horrific discovery and gasped, "Oh, my entrails are coming out!" Gentle took the panicked woman to the house of the nearest surgeon, one Mr. Mushat, but found he wasn't home. He enlisted the help of two other constables, one of whom escorted Julia to University College Hospital on Gower Street, while Gentle and the other officer took Sullivan into custody. The drunken perpetrator ranted that he was only sorry that the lover he had imagined his wife to be sleeping with hadn't been around as well, or he'd have "served them both alike."

❧

THE MAJORITY OF sick and injured people who came into University College Hospital, including Julia Sullivan, did so through the casualty and outpatient department. Very few were granted admission onto the wards. This wasn't unusual. In general, a sick person had a one-in-four chance of gaining entry onto a ward of a city hospital. In 1845, King's College Hospital treated all but 1,160 of the 17,093 people who came through its doors as outpatients. Most hospitals had a "taking-in day" designated for admitting new patients onto the wards. This might happen only once a week. In 1835, *The Times* reported an incident in which a young woman suffering from a fistula, inflammation of the brain, and consumption was turned away from Guy's Hospital in London on a Monday because taking-in day was Friday. Returning on the appropriate day, the woman arrived ten minutes late and was refused admittance because of her lack of punctuality. Dejected and seriously ill, she returned to the countryside, where she died a few days later.

In the nineteenth century, almost all the hospitals in London except the Royal Free controlled inpatient admission through a system of ticketing. One could obtain a ticket from one of the hospital's "subscribers," who had paid an annual fee in exchange for the right to recommend patients to the hospital and vote in elections of medical staff. Securing a ticket required tireless soliciting on the part of potential patients, who might spend days waiting and calling upon the servants of subscribers and begging their way into the hospital. Preference was given to acute cases. "Incurables"—people with cancer or tuberculosis, for instance—were turned away, as were people with venereal infections.

Julia Sullivan was lucky in at least one respect that evening. The life-threatening nature of her injury guaranteed her immediate attention, and although Lister had never performed an operation on his own and was woefully inexperienced when it came to treating trauma patients, it was nevertheless her great fortune that she was placed in his care. After she was rushed through the doors of the hospital on a stretcher, Lister quickly examined her lower abdomen.

Both her outer garments and her undergarments had been slashed, and the vertical cut was about two-thirds of an inch long and was wet with blood. Underneath her clothes, nearly eight inches of her intestines had slipped out of the wound.

Lister remained calm during what was a terrifying moment. After administering an anesthetic, he washed the fecal matter off the entrails with blood-warm water and gently attempted to return the intestines to their rightful place. But the young surgeon realized the opening was too small to allow this and that he would have to widen it.

Lister reached for a scalpel and cautiously enlarged the wound, upward and inward, by about three-fourths of an inch. He eased the greater part of the protrusion back into the abdominal cavity until only the knuckle of the intestine, which had been sliced by Sullivan's knife, lingered outside the wound. Proceeding very carefully, he used a fine needle and silk to stitch up the opening. He closed the wound, knotted the silk, cut off the ends, and returned the injured part of the intestine to the cavity, using the skin gash as a valve to hinder further bleeding and soiling. After Lister dealt with the gut, some red watery fluid escaped from Julia's bruised and swollen abdomen. He was happy that very "little blood had been lost, and the patient was perfectly sensible, though somewhat faint."

Returning the entrails in two stages allowed Lister time to concentrate on sewing up the wound using a single thread. His bold decision to suture Julia's gut was an extremely controversial procedure that even the most experienced surgeons often refused to undertake. Where Lister had been successful with this method, many others were not. The surgeon Andrew Ellis remarked in 1846 that "you will meet with much discrepancy of opinion when you read the various works which treat [incised intestines]." Some preferred to do nothing, keeping instead a careful watch on the situation, as in the case of the aptly named surgeon Mr. Cutler and his patient Thomas

V——, who sustained a knife wound to the gut while wrestling with a friend. When Thomas arrived at the hospital, the surgeon noted that he was suffering no significant outward bleeding and prescribed twenty drops of laudanum to the poor man writhing in pain. The next day, his bowels began to fail, and the patient's abdomen became painfully distended. Cutler ordered that the man be given an enema to ease his discomfort, but this produced no effect, so the surgeon gave him four ounces of brandy. On the third day, the patient continued in his agonized state. His skin and extremities became very cold, his pulse very faint. He was once again given an enema of senna with castor oil, which produced a small quantity of feces. Afterward, he rallied a little, only to collapse later that day and die.

Although the use of sutures was widespread at the time, stitched wounds or incisions often became infected. The risk was even higher when dealing with a punctured bowel. Most surgeons preferred to cauterize the opening with a narrow iron blade, heated on a brazier until it was red-hot. "The more slowly [the flesh] burns, the more powerful is the effect," the surgeon John Lizars remarked. If it burned deeply, the lesion could remain open for weeks or even months, healing from the inside out. The pain, of course, was excruciating, and the procedure carried with it no guarantee of survival, especially because the patient would have to convalesce on a poorly ventilated ward of a Victorian hospital crawling with bacteria and other germs.

These were the medical realities facing most people unfortunate enough to sustain an abdominal injury during the Victorian period. Lister's success with Julia Sullivan's operation was due to a combination of skill and luck. Certainly, he took his lead from hernia cases, which involved returning protrusions of the bowel back into the body. Very early in Lister's residency, Erichsen cared for a patient who had sustained a kick to the abdomen as a child and as a consequence suffered from a persistent hernia. Decades later, the hernia became swollen and painful. Erichsen was forced to cut through the man's intestines to relieve pressure in his gut before returning the bowel to its rightful place. The man seemed to recover immediately following the surgery, only to die the next day.

In addition to his observation of similar cases under Erichsen's care, it's likely that Lister had been studying the subject shortly before Julia was rushed through the doors of University College Hospital. In fact, strangulated hernias resulting from penetrating wounds were a hot topic due to the high incidences of stabbings and industrial accidents being treated in urban hospitals. George James Guthrie had written a book on the subject four years earlier, in 1847. The surgeon Benjamin Travers had also written extensively on the matter. In 1826, he described in the *Edinburgh Journal of Medical Science* a case like Julia Sullivan's. The woman in question had been brought to St. Thomas' Hospital with a self-inflicted wound to the gut that she had carried out with a razor blade. She was faint on arrival. Travers proceeded to sew up the incised part of her intestine with a silk ligature before enlarging the opening so he could return the protruding viscera to the abdominal cavity and then closed the wound with a quill suture. The patient was denied food and liquids for twenty-four hours. She continued to recover over the next few weeks until she suffered from a sudden inflammation of the bowel. As a result, the surgeon applied sixteen leeches to her abdomen and administered an enema. The wound eventually healed, and she was discharged from St. Thomas' two months after the operation.

As a medical student, Lister was familiar with the literature on these cases. And there was another reason why he might have been unusually well equipped to operate on Julia's incised gut that night. Four months earlier, *The Lancet* announced that the competition for the Fothergillian Gold Medal issued once every three years by the

Medical Society of London would focus on wounds and injuries of the abdomen and their treatment. Lister had already received several recognitions for his work at UCL, and the Fothergillian Gold Medal was one of the more prestigious awards around. Was Lister brushing up on his understanding of abdominal wounds in the hope that he might be able to enter an essay in the competition?

Although Lister's operation was a success, Julia's recovery had only just begun. Lister restricted her to a liquid diet for the remainder of her recovery to ease the pressure in her bowels. He also ordered that Julia be given a regular dose of opium, a drug that had become more popular than alcohol in the nineteenth century due to the ever-expanding British Empire. Before the Pharmacy Act of 1868 limited the sale of dangerous substances to qualified druggists, a person could buy opium from just about anyone, from barbers and confectioners to ironmongers, tobacconists, and wine merchants. Lister administered the powerful drug to patients of all ages, including children.

Over the next several weeks, Erichsen took over the case from Lister, who despite his heroic efforts in the operating theater was still a subordinate at the hospital. Like the woman at St. Thomas' Hospital, Julia began experiencing peritonitis shortly after her operation. Erichsen's treatment included the use of leeches, poultices, and fomentations to alleviate the tympanic effects of the condition. Julia finally recovered. Later in 1851, her case was twice referred to in *The Lancet*. The journal stressed the significance of Julia's recovery: "[The surgery] is of such importance . . . that we have thought it advisable to enter into greater detail than we are wont to do."

TWO MONTHS AFTER Julia Sullivan's operation, on a humid day in August, Lister boarded an omnibus to travel across the city to the Old Bailey to testify against her husband, who was on trial for attempted murder. By the mid-nineteenth century, it was not uncommon for surgeons to give evidence in court. They spoke on a wide range of matters, such as the mental health of defendants, various types of wounds, and the chemical or physiological signs of criminal poisoning, which was quickly becoming the "fashionable" way to dispose of an enemy in the Victorian period. Lister was among six people the court called upon to testify against Sullivan.

The Old Bailey was the most feared theater of justice in the country. Its fortresslike edifice was encased in a semicircular brick wall designed to prevent communication between its prisoners and the public. It sat immediately next to the notorious Newgate Prison, which had once held captive such famous personalities as Daniel Defoe, Captain Kidd, and William Penn, founder of Pennsylvania. Just in front of the two buildings was an open square where public executions took place until 1868. Thousands of spectators congregated on the day of a hanging, scrambling for a place close to the scaffold where they could witness the victim struggle against the deadly constriction of a noose. As little as two days might elapse between a guilty verdict and death for the convicted.

Charles Dickens wrote of the Old Bailey, "Nothing is so likely to strike the person who enters [the courts] for the first time, as the calm indifference with which the proceedings are conducted; every trial seems a mere matter of business." Lawyers, jury members, and court watchers lounged on hard wooden benches, reading the morning newspapers and conversing in low whispers. Some dozed off while waiting for the next case to be called. The atmosphere of nonchalance that pervaded the court could be deeply unsettling to the uninitiated. An outsider could have been forgiven if he missed the fact that the verdicts given at the Old Bailey were frequently carried out at the end of a rope.

Sullivan stood in the dock directly facing the witness box. Above him was a sounding board to amplify his voice. During the eighteenth century, a mirrored reflector was placed above the dock in order to reflect light into the faces of the accused. By Lister's time, this had been replaced with gas lighting. This measure allowed judge and jury to examine the defendants' facial expressions in order to assess the validity of their testimonies, a dubious method that led to many receiving wrongful convictions. To Sullivan's right sat the twelve members of the jury. Without leaving the room, they were expected to consult one another and arrive at a verdict within earshot of the defendant, whose fate hung in the balance. Behind and above them were the spectator galleries, where people came to watch the proceedings unfold, much as they did in the operating theater. This was an age in which matters of life and death constituted public entertainment.

The first to testify was Thomas Gentle, the police officer who attended to Julia after the stabbing. He told the court that the prisoner had been drunk when he took him into custody. In contrast, he said, the victim had been sober when she identified Jeremiah Sullivan as her attacker and was in her right mind before, during, and after the assault. Two other witnesses followed, both testifying that they had heard Sullivan threaten his wife prior to the attack.

Next, Julia herself stepped up to the witness box. Fully recovered and showing no ill effects from the injury she received, she fearlessly faced her attacker, whom she hadn't seen since the night he had stabbed her. In a lengthy deposition, Julia recalled the events of June 26. At one point, Sullivan accused her of living with another man in the hope that this would mitigate the charge of attempted murder. The court asked Julia if she had ever been unfaithful to her husband, to which she answered, "Never, in my life; he cannot bring any one to say I have been deceitful to him—he has been a murderer to me, and always was."

At last, it was Lister's turn to take the stand. He donned the muted colors of his Quaker faith. His somber demeanor gave him an air of authority that was rare for a man of his age. The young surgeon reported to the judge and jury, "I found a coil of intestine about eight inches across, comprehending, perhaps, about a yard of the small intestines, protruding from the lower part of the abdomen . . . no doubt all was done by one instrument and one stroke." The bloodied knife, which was found by Thomas Walsh, a thirteen-year-old errand boy working in the shop next to the house of the surgeon Mr. Mushat, was produced for the inspection of the court. A hush fell over the room as spectators in the public gallery leaned forward to catch a glimpse of the weapon. The prosecutor accused Sullivan of ditching the knife before Gentle and the other constable had taken him into custody. It would have been a perfect moment to do so with everyone's attention still focused on finding his wife the urgent medical care she needed. The knife was handed to Lister, who inspected it closely before confirming that its form was consistent with the type of injury Julia sustained and was therefore very likely the weapon Sullivan used to stab his wife.

Lister's testimony was damning. Sullivan was found guilty of attempted murder and sentenced to twenty years' transportation, which meant he would be banished to a penal colony in Australia. Due to the mounting pressure of London's overcrowded prisons, 162,000 convicts were transported to Australia between 1787 and 1857. Seven out of eight of these were men. Some were as young as nine, others as old as eighty. Transportation was no easy alternative to imprisonment or hanging. The convicts were first sent to hulks, or floating prisons, on the Thames. The conditions on these decommissioned, rotting ships were horrendous, and even the hospitals could not compete with them as breeding grounds for disease. Prisoners were locked in cages belowdecks in appalling surroundings. One guard remembered "seeing the shirts of the prisoners, when hung out upon the rigging, so black with vermin that the linen positively appeared to have been sprinkled over with pepper." During cholera outbreaks, the chaplain often refused to bury the dead until there was deemed to be a sufficient quantity of bloated, decomposing corpses of which to dispose. If a prisoner survived the hulks, he was shipped to Australia. One in three died on the grueling sea passage, which could take as long as eight months. If convicts behaved themselves, their sentence could be reduced by a "certificate of freedom," which would allow them to return home. The majority, however, never made it back to Britain, choosing to live out the remainder of their miserable lives in exile rather than endure the treacherous sea passage to an English port.

As horrible as banishment was, it was still better than death. Had Julia not survived, Jeremiah Sullivan would certainly have found himself dangling from the end of a noose outside Newgate Prison, a matter of days after an inevitable murder conviction. In that sense, both owed their lives to the surgeon who, when faced with the terrifying prospect of performing his first major operation entirely alone, acted quickly and decisively. It was the first of many surgical triumphs that Lister could call his own.

4.

THE ALTAR OF SCIENCE

—

Men may rise on stepping-stones
Of their dead selves to higher things.

—ALFRED, LORD TENNYSON

E VERY WEDNESDAY, THE SURGEONS and their staff assembled in
the tiny operating theater at University College Hospital. They
operated according to seniority, and orders to wipe down the
blood-soaked table between procedures were rarely issued. As Erichsen's house surgeon, Lister attended these operations, observing,
recording, assisting. It was in that modest room—with its small
instrument cupboard and solitary washbasin—that he began to
understand just how much of a lottery surgery was in the 1850s.

There were some incredibly lucky cases on these fateful Wednesdays, such as that of the young woman who was rushed into the hospital suffering from an acute disease of the larynx. On the day she arrived, Lister stood near Erichsen as he cut into the tender flesh of the woman's neck. Dark, sticky blood gushed from the incision. Erichsen frantically began slicing through the cricoid cartilage in order to make a free aperture into the air passages, but to no avail. The patient started to asphyxiate on the large quantities of fluid trapped in her chest. Her pulse slowed, and for a moment all that could be heard was the loud whistling of the air that her lungs were trying to draw into her windpipe. At that moment, Erichsen improvised something extraordinary: he clamped his mouth around the open wound in her neck and began to suck out the blood and mucus blocking her air passage. After three mouthfuls, the patient's pulse quickened, and the color returned to her cheeks. The woman survived against all odds and returned to the wards. But Lister knew that fresh dangers awaited her there. Surviving the knife was only half the battle.

The injuries and afflictions that surgeons dealt with were as varied as London's population itself. The city was ceaselessly expanding when Lister was working with Erichsen. Thousands of workers migrated to the city each year. Not only were these people living in filth due to the shortage of housing brought on by such rapid urbanization, but their jobs were both physically demanding and hazardous. All of these privations had consequences for their health. The hospital wards were clogged with people who had been maimed, blinded, suffocated, and crippled by the hazardous realities of the modernizing world.

Between 1834 and 1850, Charing Cross Hospital treated 66,000 emergencies, including 16,552 falls from scaffolds or buildings; 1,308 accidents involving steam engines, mill cogs, or cranes; 5,090 road crashes; and 2,088 burns or scalds. *The Spectator* reported that almost a third of these injuries were caused by "broken glass or porcelain, casual falls . . . lifting of weights and incautious use of spokes, hooks, knives and other domestic implements." These accidents often involved children, such as thirteen-year-old Martha Appleton, who was employed at a cotton-spinning mill as a "scavenger," which entailed picking up loose material from beneath the machinery. Overworked and undernourished, little Martha fainted one day, and her left hand was jammed in an unattended machine. She lost all five of her fingers, as well as her job. Her story was a familiar one.

During the working week, Lister encountered many cases of injury and illness brought on by poor living and working conditions. He also saw a fair share of ailments that had only recently become commonplace. There was a fifty-six-year-old painter named Mr. Larecy, for instance, who had been working between ten and fifteen hours each day since he was a young boy. He came onto the wards suffering from a severe attack of what was known as "painter's colic," a chronic intestinal disorder caused by overexposure to the lead found in paint. This was a growing problem for an industrializing nation with increasing numbers of people entering workplaces that exposed them to chemicals and metals. Even when poisonous substances like arsenic or lead were absent, the sheer amount of dust from the production and processing of steel, stone, clay, and other materials could kill a worker. It frequently took years before the damage presented itself, by which stage it was often too late. As John Thomas Arlidge—a Victorian doctor who took a keen interest in occupational medicine—observed, "Dust does not kill suddenly, but settles, year after year, a little more firmly into the lungs, until at length a case of plaster is formed. Breathing becomes more and more difficult and depressed, and finally ceases." Bronchitis, pneumonia, and a variety of other respiratory diseases put many of the working class into an early grave.

Lister also observed the effects of diet on the health of the city's laborers. Besides consuming large quantities of beer on a daily basis, nearly all of his patients ate huge amounts of cheap meat but very few vegetables or portions of fruit. Over the summer, two people came onto Lister's wards with sunken eyes, ghostly pale skin, and tooth loss—the telltale signs of scurvy. Doctors didn't yet understand that scurvy was brought on by a lack of vitamin C, which the human body is unable to synthesize for itself. In fact, many practitioners believed it was caused by a lack of mineral salt in the body. In keeping with this line of thought, Lister treated both patients with nitrate of potash, a mineral that many in the medical community wrongly believed could cure the disease.

If the low quality of the poor's food was an obvious daily problem, then the long-term repercussions of another human imperative were slightly more insidious. Over time, Lister developed a practiced eye for the varying signs of sexually transmitted diseases. Many of the patients whom he treated were afflicted with the pox (syphilis). Before the twentieth century, syphilis was an incurable and ultimately fatal disease. Those suffering from it often turned to surgeons because a majority of their work at this time dealt not with operative surgery but with external afflictions. The symptoms syphilis engendered worsened over time. In addition to the unsightly skin ulcers that pockmarked the body in the later stages of the disease, many victims endured paralysis, blindness, dementia, and "saddle nose," a grotesque deformity that occurs when the bridge of the nose caves into the face. (Syphilis was so common that "no nose clubs" sprang up all over London. One newspaper reported that "an eccentric gentleman, having taken a fancy to see a large party of noseless persons, invited every one thus afflicted, whom he met in the streets, to dine on a certain day at a tavern, where he formed them into a brotherhood." The man, who assumed the alias of Mr. Crampton for these clandestine parties, entertained his noseless friends every month for a year until his death, at which time the group "unhappily dissolved.")

Many treatments for syphilis involved the use of mercury, which could be administered in the form of an ointment, a steam bath, or a pill. Unfortunately, the side effects could be as painful and as terrifying as the disease itself. Most patients who underwent extensive treatments experienced multiple tooth loss, ulcerations, and neurological damage. Frequently, people died from mercury poisoning before they died of the disease itself.

At University College Hospital, a fifty-six-year-old Irish laborer named Matthew Kelly had been admitted after suffering from three severe falls, which he feared were caused by "the falling sickness," or epilepsy. Lister, however, was suspicious of the painful spots on his thighs and wondered if there could be another cause of his fits. Given the man's sexual history and "strong inclination to venery," Lister suspected that Kelly was actually experiencing incipient cerebritis, or the last stages of syphilis, which can include seizures that appear epileptic in nature. Because this disease was so little understood, there was not much Lister could do for Kelly, and he was eventually released from the hospital after being deemed incurable.

It was not the only occasion on which Lister had to discharge unwell patients, sometimes endangering the health of those with whom they might come into contact. Another case involved a twenty-one-year-old shoemaker named James Chappell, who was admitted onto the hospital's wards during the summer of 1851. He had contracted both syphilis and gonorrhea several years earlier and had been in and out of hospitals ever since. Lister noted that although the young man was unmarried, he had been engaged in sexual activity since he was fifteen. Lister recorded in his casebooks that Chappell "formed a connexion with a female, and sometimes at this early age had connexion 3 or 4 times a day." The most pressing concern for Chappell was not, however, the consequences of his irrepressible libido. What had brought him to Lister's ward was a hacking cough that was accompanied by white discharge tinged with blood, sometimes amounting to as much as one and a half pints. The diagnosis was plain: first-stage phthisis, or pulmonary tuberculosis—a respiratory disease for which there was no cure in the 1850s. Hospital policy dictated that incurables not be admitted, and so Lister sent Chappell back out into the general population. The medical community did not yet know that tuberculosis is a highly infectious disease. The fact that Chappell was forced to sleep in the same room with five or six of his shop mates leaves one wondering how many other people he infected. Such was life for the typical Victorian worker who came to frequent the wards of London's hospitals.

WHILE URBANIZATION took a toll on the health of its working class, Britain was eagerly celebrating its seemingly unassailable status as a global mercantile powerhouse. In the summer of 1851, the city swelled with millions of visitors who had come to see the Great Exhibition in Hyde Park, which signaled to the nation that technology was the key to a better future.

Sparkling amid the trees was the Crystal Palace, built by the garden designer Joseph Paxton as a showcase for wonders of industry from around the world. The enormous building was modeled on Paxton's glass greenhouses. Fashioned from nearly one million square feet of glass, the Crystal Palace was 1,851 feet long—a number deliberately chosen to reflect the year of the exhibition—and it boasted six times more floor space than St. Paul's Cathedral. During its construction, contractors tested the building's structural integrity by ordering three hundred compliant laborers to jump up and down on the flooring, and by having troops of soldiers march around its bays.

When the exhibition opened, there were approximately 100,000 objects from more than fifteen thousand contributors on display, among them a printing machine that could turn out five thousand copies of *The Illustrated London News* in an hour; "tangible ink" that produced raised characters on paper for the blind; and a handful of velocipedes, the predecessor of the modern bicycle, with pedals and cranks on the front axle. The biggest exhibit by far was a massive hydraulic press, which could be operated by just one man, even though each metal tube weighed 1,144 tons. There was also the world's first major installation of public flushing toilets, designed by the Victorian sanitary engineer George Jennings. Some 827,280 people paid one penny to use the facilities during the exhibition, which gave rise to the popular euphemism "spending a penny." But such a luxury would not ameliorate the squalor of Britain's poorest households for many years to come.

There were scientific and medical novelties too, the more practical of which would find their way into the hospitals of Britain. An artificial leech that looked like a miniature bicycle pump was meant to expel "matters and humours from the body" and infuse "animating substances through the skin." There were prosthetic hands, arms, and legs that promised to restore an amputee's ability to grasp objects, ride a horse, or dance. One exhibitor from Paris showcased a complete model of the human body made from seventeen hundred parts that included replicas of bones, muscles, veins, and spinal nerves. The five-foot-nine dummy even had crystalline lenses in its eyes, which could be removed to reveal optic nerves and membranes underneath.

The curious traveled from all over the world to marvel at the contraptions that promised to make everyday life easier, faster, and more convenient. One woman walked 247 miles from Penzance on the southwest tip of England to attend the fair. In a letter to her father, the celebrated novelist Charlotte Brontë wrote of the Great Exhibition, "It is a wonderful place—vast, strange, new and impossible to describe. Its grandeur does not consist in one thing, but in the unique assemblage of all things. Whatever human industry has created, you find there." The Victorians had come to worship at the altar of science, and they had not been disappointed. By the time the Great Exhibition closed on October 11, more than six million people had visited the park, including Joseph Lister and his father, Joseph Jackson, whose nephew had displayed a microscope that was honored with an award by the exhibition organizers.

The true value of the microscope continued to be debated and disputed within the wider medical community in the 1850s. And yet Lister persisted with his research. After the fair had ended, he spent an inordinate amount of time poring over microscope slides that he had prepared. Anything and everything he could lay his hands on ended up under the lens. One afternoon in late autumn, he watched as an amorphous mass of bloody tissue danced before his eyes. Lister squinted into the ocular lens of his microscope before turning the tiny brass dial on the sleek instrument to adjust the focus. Suddenly, the tumor that he and Erichsen had excised from a patient earlier that day popped into view, each cell outlined with perfect clarity. Lister studied the image for a few minutes before he began to sketch the tumor on a pad of paper. He produced dozens of images like this, some of them in such startling detail that he was able to use them as teaching aids decades later.

Even when he toured the country on vacations, his mind was constantly engaged with the natural world around him. Lister sketched muscle tissues from the leg of a spider and the corneal cells from the eye of a boiled lobster. He sliced open starfish he had trapped during a trip to Torquay—a seaside town on the English Channel—and delighted in observing their odd geometric shapes magnified under the lens. Writing to his father, he boasted, "I even saw . . . a valve in the middle of the upper part of the heart alternately open and close at each pulse." After he had caught a lamprey in the Thames, he cut into the silvery body and extracted the eel's brain late at night in his room. Using a camera lucida—an optical device that allowed an artist to trace images projected onto sheets of paper—Lister was able to sketch in precise detail the creature's medulla cells that he had observed with his microscope.

Lister found an ally for his microscopic research in his professor of physiology. William Sharpey—then in his early fifties—looked as though he were permanently squinting, which seemed apt given the amount of time the man spent peering down the lens of his own microscope. The hair on the top of the Scotsman's head had thinned considerably by the time Lister came under his tutelage in 1851, though he tried to compensate for the loss by keeping the sides conspicuously bushy. Sharpey was the first to teach a complete course of lectures on physiology, a subject that had traditionally been treated as an appendage to anatomy. This later earned him the title "the Father of Modern Physiology." He was both an intellectual and a physical giant. When demonstrating to his class how to work a spirometer—an instrument devised to measure the capacity of air in the lungs—he filled each cell of the device so effortlessly that he observed afterward, "This instrument seems to have been designed for people of ordinary development."

Lister took to Sharpey immediately. He saw in him a man similar to his own father. The physiology professor valued experiment and observation over authority, a characteristic that was unusual in its day. Later in life, Lister reminisced,

> As a student at University College I was greatly attracted by
> Dr. Sharpey's lectures, which inspired me with a love of
> physiology that has never left me. My father, whose
> labours . . . had raised the compound microscope from
> little better than a scientific toy to the powerful engine for
> investigation which it then already was, had equipped me

with a first-rate instrument of that kind and I employed it
with keen interest in verifying the details of histology
brought before us by our great master.

Spurred on by Sharpey's enthusiasm, Lister began to observe as
much human tissue under the microscope as he could acquire. His
sketches reveal intricate details of everything from human skin to
the cells of a cancerous tongue, which had been cut out of a patient.
Lister also created full-color clinical paintings of patients he encountered at the hospital. This was the only method of recording case
histories visually before the advent of color photography. In one such
painting, Lister portrayed a man leaning back, his arm resting on a
chair. His sleeve is rolled up, and his skin is pockmarked with angry
sores, probably venereal in nature.

Lister wasn't content with just being an observer. He also conducted his own experiments, building upon the work of the Italian
priest and physiologist Lazzaro Spallanzani, who was the first to
correctly describe how the process of mammalian reproduction relied on the union of spermatozoon and ovum. In 1784, Spallanzani
developed a technique for artificially inseminating dogs, as well as
frogs and even fish. Taking his cue from Spallanzani, Lister took the
sperm of a cockerel and tried to artificially fertilize the egg of a
chicken outside the body of the bird—but it didn't work out. (It
would take another hundred years before a doctor successfully repeated this experiment in a human. In 1884, the American physician
William Pancoast injected sperm from his "best-looking" student
into an anesthetized woman—without her knowledge—whose husband had been deemed infertile. Nine months later, she gave birth
to a healthy baby. Pancoast eventually told her husband what he had
done, but the two men decided to spare the woman the truth.
Pancoast's experiment remained a secret for twenty-five years. After
his death in 1909, the donor—a man ironically named Dr. Addison

Davis Hard—confessed to the underhanded deed in a letter to *Medical World*.)

In 1852, Lister made his first major contribution to science using the microscope when he turned his attention to the human eye after obtaining a portion of "fresh blue iris" from Wharton Jones, the university's professor of ophthalmology. Lister was interested in the debate concerning the nature of the tissue in the constrictor and dilator muscles of the iris. The Swiss physiologist Albert von Kölliker had recently described this tissue as comprising smooth muscle cells, like the kind found in the stomach, the blood vessels, or the bladder. The actions of this type of muscle are involuntary. Kölliker's discovery was in opposition to the view upheld by one of England's most eminent ophthalmologists, William Bowman, who believed that the tissue was striped (or striated), which would make the muscle's movements voluntary.

Lister carefully teased portions of tissue from the iris, which had only been excised from the patient four hours earlier. He placed the sample under the microscope and studied it over the next five and a half hours, sketching each individual cell using the camera lucida. During the course of his research into the matter, Lister examined irises taken from five additional surgical patients at University College Hospital, as well as irises from a horse, a cat, a rabbit, and a guinea pig. What he found confirmed Kölliker's theory that the iris is in fact composed of smooth muscle fibers arranged as both constrictors and dilators and that their actions are indeed involuntary. Lister published his conclusions in the *Quarterly Journal of Microscopical Science*. His research stood him apart from so many in his profession who continued to view the microscope as superfluous to the practice of medicine.

Lister's experiments were undoubtedly considered esoteric by many of the faculty and students alike because they could offer little to the advancement of surgery in the 1850s. And yet Lister persisted.

Progress in the form of urbanization and industrialization came at a human cost, but progress in the form of science might provide answers to growing problems within the hospitals. Perhaps the microscope would unlock secrets about the human body that could one day lead to changes in therapeutics.

—

A FEW MONTHS LATER, another patient on Erichsen's wards fell ill with an infectious disease. This time the deadly culprit was hospital gangrene, the most virulent of the "big four" that made up hospitalism. Some doctors called the condition a malignant or "phagedenic" ulcer, the latter deriving from Greek and meaning "to eat away." The Scottish surgeon John Bell wrote about the horror of hospital gangrene after treating numerous patients who had died from it. In the first stage, "the wound swells, the skin retracts . . . the cellular membrane is melted down into a foetid mucus, and the fascia is exposed." As the disease progresses, the wound enlarges and the skin is eaten away, exposing the deep layer of muscles and bone. The patient goes into shock and begins experiencing intense nausea and diarrhea as the body tries to expel the poison from within. The pain is excruciating, and alas, delirium is rare. The patient remains conscious throughout the whole miserable ordeal. Bell wrote, "The cries of the sufferers are the same in the night as in the day-time; they are exhausted in the course of a week and die: or if they survive, and the ulcers continue to eat down and disjoin the muscles, the great vessels are at last exposed and eroded, and they bleed to death."

The first English descriptions of the affliction come from late eighteenth-century naval surgeons, who witnessed outbreaks of it in the damp, cramped quarters of the king's fleet. Isolated on the high seas, the sailors could do nothing to contain its spread once it appeared, and the sickly sweet smell of rotting flesh would soon pervade the already fetid air belowdecks. In the summer of 1799, one surgeon saw a sailor punched in the ear during a brawl. He suffered a slight wound from the blow. Within days, however, an ulcer had appeared that devoured one side of the man's face and neck, exposing his trachea and the inside of his throat before killing him.

Hundreds of stories like this abound. On the HMS *Saturn*, a malignant ulcer appeared on the tip of a seaman's penis. After several days of agonizing pain during which the wound blackened and festered, the organ finally fell off. The surgeon on board reported that the "whole length of the urethra to the bulb sloughed away, and also the scrotum, leaving the testes and spermatic vessels barely covered with cellular substance." As if the inevitable outcome needed underlining, the surgeon added, "He died."

When it came to these festering, flesh-eating ulcers, Bell advised that patients be removed from the hospital as quickly as possible: "Without the circle of infected walls men are safe." Anything was better than "this house of death," as Bell put it. Let the surgeon "lay them in a school-room, a church, on a dung-hill, or in a stable." Others agreed: "This hospital gangrene . . . no doubt depends on the unwholesome atmosphere exciting preternatural irritability, and the treatment, therefore, essentially requires removal from the sphere of this deleterious influence."

Erichsen did not differ in his thinking. He too subscribed to the long-held belief that hospital gangrene was caused by a corruption in the air. But isolating the afflicted from other patients could be difficult. When outbreaks occurred, the problem was as much political as it was medical. Wards had to be shut. Admissions had to be halted. Everyone from the hospital administrators to the surgeons themselves scrambled to contain its relentless spread.

When Lister saw filmy discharge seeping through a patient's dressings one day in 1852, this must have been on his mind. As he peeled back the damp bandages, he was met with a powerful odor emanating from a rotting, ulcerating wound. An epidemic of hospital gangrene soon swept Erichsen's wards as a result of this single patient. Lister was quickly put in charge of carrying out treatment on the infected—a task that reflects just how far he had come in his residency to be trusted with such important work.

At the height of the outbreak, Lister observed something peculiar. He routinely scraped away the brown pultaceous slough from patients' infected wounds while they were anesthetized. He then applied mercury pernitrate, a highly caustic and toxic solution, to them. Afterward, he recorded in his notebook: "As a rule . . . a perfectly healthy granulating sore was disclosed which healed kindly under ordinary dressings." Only in one case—that of a "very stout woman, in whom the disease attacked an enormous wound of the forearm"—had the mercury pernitrate not worked. Instead, the infection spread with "astonishing rapidity" over the entire sore, and eventually the arm had to be amputated by Erichsen. But before the operation, Lister cleaned out the wound and washed her arm thoroughly with soap and water. The amputation was a success, and the stump healed perfectly—a fact Lister attributed to his own efforts to sanitize the arm beforehand.

Lister's curiosity had been piqued. Why was it that a majority of the ulcers healed when they were debrided and cleaned with the caustic solution? Although he didn't dismiss the idea that miasma could be partly to blame, he wasn't convinced that the foul air was entirely responsible for what was happening on the wards of University College Hospital. Something in the wound itself had to be at fault—not just the air around the patient. From the pus that he had scraped out of the infected wounds, he carefully prepared microscopic slides to examine under the lens. The implications of what he saw would take root in his mind and eventually make him question an entire belief system upheld by no less a figure than his superior and mentor, John Eric Erichsen.

He later recorded, "I examined microscopically the slough from one of the sores, and I made a sketch of some bodies of pretty uniform size which I imagined might be the *materies morbi* [morbid substances] . . . the idea that it was probably of parasitic nature was at that early period already present in my mind."

Lister's revelation inspired him to conduct broader investigations into the causes of hospital infection. Despite his reenergized commitment to surgery, however, he remained unsure of his career path. Having come across a variety of medical cases during his house surgeoncy, he flirted with the idea of becoming a physician. After completing his residency under Erichsen, Lister accepted an appointment as clinical clerk (the equivalent of a dresser on the medical side) to the senior physician Dr. Walter H. Walshe at University College Hospital. Lister's nephew Rickman John Godlee later said that "the allurements of medicine seem to have been even stronger than those of surgery" at this time.

During his final year at UCL, Lister was awarded several distinctions and gold medals that elevated him above his peers. The prizes were prestigious and fiercely contested among medical students at the university and among those studying at London's teaching hospitals. He won the Longridge Prize for "Greatest Proficiency . . . for Medical Honours and credible performance of duties of offices at the Hospital" and was awarded the considerable sum of forty pounds because of it. He also received a gold medal and a scholarship worth a hundred pounds for the results of his second examination in medicine. Lister began to overcome his shyness, due in part to the recognition of his talents and his newfound authority among the student body. His friend and fellow lodger Sampson Gamgee wrote to Lister, "Had it not been for you, University College would have been a nonentity at the examinations for honours at the University, whereas it now stands second school in London, placing Guy's first and St. George's third."

Even so, not everyone was enamored with Lister's mercurial, questing mind. When the time came to graduate, he was placed last on the honors list for physiology and comparative anatomy. His professor William Carpenter cited the reason for this slight in a letter to him: "I think it as well to let you know the reason why I found it requisite to place you there. . . . As answers to my questions, your papers were so defective, that if it had not been for the amount of original observation of which they bore evidence, I could not have placed you in the honours list at all." Lister was irritated by Carpenter's decision. As he wrote to his brother-in-law Rickman Godlee (later, father of Rickman John Godlee), "I care but little comparatively for this, for I find from conversing with him that it is just a question of whether you have or have not read his book."

It was true that Lister wasn't disposed to accept something simply because his professors told him it was so. One of the more interesting cases that came his way as a house surgeon—and one that best demonstrates his inability to accept the authority of his superiors as the final word—involved a sixty-four-year-old man with hepatitis. In addition to an excess of biliary matter in the man's urine, Lister noted that it contained too much sugar and wondered whether the latter was a normal constituent of the bile. He turned to the recently appointed professor of chemistry at UCL for answers but found he was not prepared to give him a clear one. Instead of letting the matter rest, Lister obtained bile from two different sheep and applied sulfate of copper and caustic potash to both samples. In neither experiment was there any evidence of sugar, which led Lister to conclude that his patient's present condition was in fact unusual. He won another gold medal for his research on the case.

At the end of 1852, Lister sat for his examinations at the Royal

College of Surgeons and became fully qualified to practice surgery. Still, he vacillated, unable to make a final commitment to the profession. In February 1853, he returned to Dr. Walshe's side, this time as a physician's assistant. His hesitancy to enter surgical practice by extending his medical studies was facilitated by his father's financial support. Partly as a consequence of coming last on the honors list for physiology and comparative anatomy, he remained diffident and doubtful. Taking a post as a fully fledged surgeon meant accepting complete responsibility for those under his care. Perhaps he fretted about what harm he might do to his future patients when confronted by obscure and rare manifestations of diseases.

Underneath the outward indecision, Lister's scientific curiosity remained steadfast and undiminished. He continued to conduct experiments and carry out his own dissections. The microscope enabled him to probe the secrets of the human body more deeply than he or the overwhelming majority of his predecessors, peers, and superiors ever had before. And there was still the question of those microbes that he detected under the lens after the outbreak of hospital gangrene on Erichsen's wards. What exactly were they, and how were they linked to what was happening to patients on the wards of the city's largest hospitals?

Professor Sharpey, always the keen observer, recognized that Lister was drifting and suggested that he spend a year touring Continental medical schools. There, Lister would learn more about recent advances made in medicine and surgery, as Sharpey himself had done decades earlier when he traipsed around Europe. Paris—with its welcoming wards, lectures on emerging clinical specialties, numerous private courses, and countless opportunities for dissection—should top Lister's itinerary, in Sharpey's opinion. But first, he wanted his pupil to spend a month in Scotland with his good friend James Syme, the renowned professor of clinical surgery at the University of Edinburgh and fourth cousin to the great Robert Liston, now very well known for his work with ether. Sharpey suspected that Syme would find in Lister an enthusiastic student eager to participate in the investigations that the two men were conducting into the nature of inflammation and the circulation of blood. He also believed that Lister would find in Syme an inspirational mentor.

And so, in September 1853, Lister boarded a train to "Auld Reekie" (or "Old Smokey"), Scotland's capital city, for what was intended to be a short stay.

5.

THE NAPOLEON OF SURGERY

—

**Were I to place a man of proper talents, in the most
direct road for becoming truely *great* in his profession,
I would chuse a good practical Anatomist, and put
him into a large hospital to attend the
sick and dissect the dead.**

—WILLIAM HUNTER

THE DEEP BAGS UNDERNEATH Professor James Syme's eyes were
indicative of the endless hours he spent inside the operating theater of Edinburgh's Royal Infirmary. He was short and stout, but
otherwise unremarkable in his appearance. His fashion choices were
singularly unbecoming, consisting of a jumbled mixture of oversized
clothes that rarely changed from day to day. His habitual apparel was
a black long-tailed coat with a stiff high collar and a checkered cravat
tied tightly around the neck. Like the promising surgeon from Lon-

don whom he was about to meet, Syme had a slight stutter, which plagued him his entire life.

Despite his small stature, Syme was a giant of his profession by the time Lister traveled to see him. His colleagues called him "the Napoleon of Surgery," a reputation that the fifty-four-year-old had acquired through his Herculean attempts to simplify traumatic procedures over the last twenty-five years of his career. Syme despised crude instruments like the hand-cranked chain saw and eschewed difficult methods when straightforward ones would suffice. Economy of time and technique was something Syme tried to achieve with nearly every form of operation he undertook. This attitude was mirrored in the characteristic brevity with which he spoke. Syme's former pupil John Brown said of his great teacher that he "never unnecessarily wasted a word, a drop of ink, or of blood."

Syme's fame was largely attributable to his groundbreaking development of an amputation at the ankle joint—a procedure that still bears his name and is performed by surgeons today. Prior to his innovative technique, surgeons amputated below the knee for compound injuries and for incurable diseases of the foot, with dire effects upon a person's mobility. This was often done because it was assumed that the long stump would be a nuisance and that the patient would not be able to walk on it. Syme's method made it possible for the patient to bear weight on the ankle stump, which was a remarkable advancement in surgery, and his method was also easier and faster than amputating below the knee.

Like many surgeons who were trained before the dawn of anesthetics, Syme was lightning-fast—as was his cousin Robert Liston. He once removed a leg at the hip joint in approximately one minute, a feat made even more extraordinary by the fact that neither he nor any other surgeon in Scotland had ever before performed this type of procedure. Of course, the operation was not without complications. When Syme made the first cut into the thighbone, just under the socket, a resounding crack could be heard throughout the operating theater. He quickly removed the leg, and his assistant relaxed his grip in order to release the arteries that needed tying off. Syme recalled the horror that followed:

> Had it not been for thorough seasoning in scenes of dreadful haemorrhage, I certainly should have been startled. . . . It seemed indeed, at first sight, as if the vessels which supplied so many large and crossing jets of arterial blood could never all be closed. It may be imagined that we did not spend much time in admiring this alarming spectacle; a single instant was sufficient to convince us that the patient's safety required all our expedition, and in the course of a few minutes haemorrhage was effectually restrained by the application of ten or twelve ligatures.

He would later call the procedure the "greatest and bloodiest operation in surgery."

Syme was fearless. When other surgeons refused to operate, the Scotsman was at hand with his knife poised. In 1828, a man named Robert Penman approached Syme in desperation. Eight years earlier, he had developed a bony, fibrous tumor in his lower jaw. At the time, it was about the size of a hen's egg. A local surgeon excised the teeth embedded in the growth, but the tumor continued to grow. When that procedure failed, Penman consulted Liston, who had recently made a name for himself by removing a forty-five-pound scrotal tumor from a patient at the Edinburgh Infirmary. Upon seeing Penman's bloated and swollen face, however, even the indomitable Liston blanched. The size and position of the tumor, he thought, made it impossible to operate. This refusal to act was tantamount to a death sentence from a surgeon who usually embraced difficult cases. If Liston wouldn't operate, who would?

Penman's condition worsened until he reached a point where eating and breathing became extremely difficult. The tumor now weighed over four and a half pounds and obscured most of his lower face. So Penman sought out Syme, who at the age of twenty-nine was already known for his maverick approach to surgery.

On the day of the operation, Penman was seated upright in a chair, with his arms and legs restrained. Because neither ether nor chloroform had yet been discovered, Penman was administered no anesthetic. The patient steadied himself as Syme stepped forward, knife in hand. Most jaw tumors were gouged out during this time, beginning at the center of the growth and extending to the periphery. Syme had a different approach in mind. He proceeded to cut into the unaffected part of the man's lower jawbone, in order to remove the tumor and some of the healthy tissue around it, and ensure that it was completely eradicated. For twenty-four excruciating minutes, Syme hacked away at the bony growth, dropping slices of tumor and jawbone with a sickening rattle into a bucket at his feet. It was incredible to those watching how anyone could endure such a horrific ordeal. And yet, against all odds, Penman survived.

Long after the operation, Syme bumped into his former patient on the street and was surprised to see that the scarring on his face was minimal. His receding chin was concealed by a luxuriant beard. Anyone looking at Penman, Syme concluded with satisfaction, would never guess that he had undergone such a traumatic procedure.

It was operations like the one done on Penman that gained Syme his reputation as one of the most daring surgeons of his generation. On a dreary day in September 1853, Joseph Lister arrived in Edinburgh to meet this surgical pioneer. He clutched the letter of introduction penned by his UCL mentor Professor Sharpey. The city was geographically smaller than London but more densely populated. Although overcrowding was a problem for most industrializing cities in Britain, Edinburgh's claustrophobic living conditions were compounded by housing shortages in the 1850s and by the thousands of Irish immigrants pouring into the city, seeking refuge from the devastation caused by the potato famine, which had only ended two years earlier.

In one district of Edinburgh, there was an average of twenty-five inhabitants living in each house. Over a third of these households occupied single-room homes, typically no bigger than fourteen by eleven feet. Many houses were packed tightly together in narrow enclosed courtyards. The twelfth-century city walls, built to protect Edinburgh's residents, constrained the outward expansion of the Old Town. As a consequence, houses grew upward, reaching dangerous heights at a time when building regulations were far from rigorous. The district's rickety structures could easily exceed ten stories, each level protruding and looming over the one before, so that the tops of these ramshackle buildings blocked out the sunlight. Those who lived on the ground floors were the poorest residents. They were surrounded by cattle and by open sewers that overflowed with human excrement just outside their front doors.

Within these quarters, crime rates soared in parallel with the growing number of inhabitants. More than fifteen thousand people were brought before the police for various offenses the year Lister arrived. Their crimes ranged from theft and begging to "allowing chimneys to take fire." Of those miscreants apprehended, thousands were charged with physical assault and public drunkenness. Punishments were meted out, often arbitrarily, without due process. Some offenders received a mere admonishment for their crimes, while others were imprisoned, whipped, or executed. A large proportion of these delinquents were children under the age of twelve, many of whom were subsequently sent to "Ragged Schools"—charitable organizations that provided free education for destitute youngsters.

The slums festered in the Old Town like weeping sores. The absence of conveniences, such as clean water and toilets, made for an atmosphere that was, according to one resident of Edinburgh, "foully tainted, and rendered almost unendurable by its loathsomeness at those periods when offal and nuisance require to be deposited on the streets." The filth and squalor that resulted from a mass of humanity being crammed into a small area created a perfect incubator for the growth of virulent diseases like typhus, tuberculosis, and relapsing fever.

Underneath this decrepit facade, Edinburgh pulsated with a dark energy. At the time Lister set foot onto its railway platform, the city had already established itself as a world leader in surgery, albeit one tainted by scandal and murder. It had been only twenty-five years since the infamous William Burke and William Hare had skulked around the streets of Edinburgh, looking for their next victim to accost. Over the course of ten months, the pair had strangled sixteen people and sold their suspiciously fresh corpses to Robert Knox, a surgeon running his own private anatomy school in the city who turned a blind eye to the duo's cagey activities. (Burke and Hare were eventually apprehended after one of their victims was recognized by a spectator in the dissection theater. Fearing for his life, Hare turned king's evidence and testified against his partner. He was pardoned for his cooperation, while Burke alone was left to swing from the end of a rope. In a poetic twist of fate, the murderer's body was later dissected publicly, with hundreds of people in attendance. He was flayed meticulously, and his skin was used to make various macabre trinkets, including pocketbooks, which were hawked to a delighted, bloodthirsty public.)

The atrocities perpetrated by Burke and Hare sprang from the lucrative trade that supplied fresh corpses to anatomy schools around

Britain in the early decades of the nineteenth century, when the only bodies that could be legally obtained for dissection were those of hanged murderers. With the proliferation of private medical schools, there simply weren't enough bodies to go around. As a result, the city was crawling with body snatchers, or "resurrectionists" as they were sometimes called. They worked under the cloak of darkness in the dead of winter, when the natural process of decomposition was slowed by the frigid Scottish weather. Using wooden spades and iron hooks, they dug a small hole at the head of each grave, broke apart the lid of the coffin, and dragged the corpse out. The men might steal as many as six bodies in a single night and often worked in small gangs that fought each other for a monopoly over the cadaver trade.

So rife was the problem that drastic measures were taken to protect the dead in graveyards around Edinburgh. The bereaved placed mortsafes—or iron grilles—over burial plots to protect departed loved ones. They capped the surrounding walls with loose stones, which made them nearly impossible to scale without creating a disturbance. Groundskeepers defended churchyards by setting up spring guns and primitive land mines. Local people organized "cemetery clubs" and held vigil by new graves for weeks until the body therein was too decomposed to be of any use to anatomy schools. In one instance, a father grieving the recent loss of his child enclosed a "small box, [with] some deathful apparatus, communicating by means of wires, with the four corners, to be fastened to the top of the coffin." As the child was lowered into the ground, he threw gunpowder into this rudimentary piece of ordnance so that "the hidden machinery [was] put into a state of readiness for execution."

By 1853, the body snatchers' nefarious activities had ceased throughout Britain due to the passing of a law that made it legal to dissect the unclaimed bodies of the poor, thus giving medical practitioners access to a large supply of corpses. But Lister's new superiors—the very men who taught at the university and would soon welcome him to Edinburgh—were products of that bygone era. Even the late Robert Liston had metaphorical dirt on his hands from his time teaching in Auld Reekie. At the height of the corpse trade, he would send his band of body snatchers to invade the territories of the gangs his peers had employed, leading to irreparable rifts between the competing anatomists.

The unpalatable truth was that without the body snatchers and the thousands of corpses they had procured for anatomists during previous decades, Edinburgh would not have established its enviable global reputation for trailblazing surgery. Without this status, it is unlikely that Lister would have gone out of his way to travel there to meet Professor Syme as a prelude to setting out on his Continental tour to visit Europe's medical institutes.

Indeed, Lister might have thought twice about a Scottish hiatus if he had known more of the Royal Infirmary's combative professional environment. In a letter to his father explaining his decision to go to Edinburgh, he wrote, "I shall not have, as in London, to fight with jealous rivals, and contend or join ingloriously with quacks. . . . I am by disposition very averse to quarreling and contending with others, in fact, I doubt if I could do it." But Joseph Lister—the shy, reserved young man entirely unaccustomed to conflict at this point in his life—was about to enter the lion's den.

At the center of much of the infirmary's conflict was Syme himself, who often evinced a dark side to his genius. He was volatile and had an unnatural inclination to nurture lifelong grudges. When the obstetrician James Y. Simpson suggested in a pamphlet that surgeons use a procedure he had devised called acupressure to control surgical hemorrhaging, Syme stormed into the operating theater, pulled out his knife, and proceeded to shred the document before a crowd of spectators. "There, gentlemen, is what acupressure is worth."

Even when his adversaries attempted reconciliation, Syme's temper and pride were frequently obstacles. In one instance, his colleague James Miller—with whom Syme had been quarreling for years due to his close friendship with Simpson, the advocate of acupressure—decided it was time to bury the hatchet. Miller had lately fallen ill and realized he would soon die. He went to visit Syme at his home in 1864. When he entered, he found the petulant surgeon standing in front of a roaring fireplace, his hands clasped behind his back. Miller said he had come to bid Syme a final goodbye and offered his hand in rapprochement. Syme looked coolly at the frail man before him and, without extending his own hand in return, replied, "Huh, so you've come to apologise, have you? Well! I forgive ye." Miller left without another word from his old rival.

Syme's quarrels were both a hindrance and a boon to his career. He fell out with Liston, with whom he had been working closely ever since he began practicing surgery. The feud seemed to evolve from a series of small disagreements coupled with a growing professional rivalry between the cousins. Liston scorned the use of the tourniquet, for example, preferring to use his left arm to stanch the flow of blood, while the less physically imposing Syme vocally opposed such primitive methods. The animosity between the two men reached a tipping point in 1829, when Syme applied for a surgeoncy at the Edinburgh Royal Infirmary, where Liston was working. Syme was turned down for the position because the hospital managers anticipated a war between the two men breaking out on the wards and disturbing the convalescents.

Syme didn't expend too much time or energy feeling sorry for himself. In that same year, he bought Minto House, a derelict mansion on Chambers Street that he planned to turn into his own private hospital. It was a brave move for a man who wasn't exactly wealthy. Syme converted the property into a public hospital with twenty-four beds. While trying to collect funds to support his endeavor, he circulated a subscription book among the city's wealthy people, who might have been able to support the project. When the book fell into Liston's hands, he inscribed within it, "Don't support quackery and humbug."

Despite Liston's churlishness, Minto House became a roaring success. Over the course of three years, Syme oversaw eight thousand cases and performed more than a thousand operations there. These included major amputations, excisions of elbows and knees, and mastectomies for "scirrhous breasts." And so when the chair of clinical surgery at the University of Edinburgh became vacant in 1833, Syme considered himself an ideal candidate given his newfound experience running a private hospital. Liston also applied for the position, but the younger cousin finally won the day.

Six years later, Liston reached out to Syme. He had now moved to London to take up an equivalent post at UCL and in due time would perform his historic operation with ether, witnessed by Joseph Lister as a medical student. In his letter to his estranged cousin, Liston spoke of his desire to bring about a reconciliation and asked Syme in medical jargon to "tell me that you wish to have our grievances and sores not plastered but firmly cicatrised." He ended his appeal with the words "I am not so bad as you believe me to be." Syme accepted the olive branch and mended the relationship.

There was no doubt that Syme had found his niche in Edinburgh. The small surgical community there was rife with feuds, rumors, and jealousy. It seemed that every surgeon was pitted against every other, at one point or another. Indeed, at times, Edinburgh could be even more febrile than London, where a surgeon once fought a duel over a medical dispute.

LISTER TOOK UP temporary lodging on South Frederick Street in the newer part of Edinburgh shortly after his arrival. The weather in September, though quite mild, was invariably depressing. Swollen rain clouds hung heavily in the sky most days, casting shadows over the city and engendering a seemingly inescapable dankness. He only intended to stay a month before heading off to sunnier pastures on his tour of Europe. Once he settled in, he presented his letter of introduction to Syme, who welcomed him warmly into the city's surgical community.

Syme oversaw three wards at the Royal Infirmary. To Lister, the hospital was a marvel. With 228 beds, it was more than twice as large as London's University College Hospital. It was massive by nineteenth-century standards. When first built in 1729, it offered beds for only four patients. In 1741, a new building was erected at High School Yards (later known as Infirmary Street). Over time, the hospital expanded—once in 1832 and again in 1853. Eventually, the Royal Infirmary would dominate the entire area situated between Drummond Street and High School Yards. The Royal Infirmary was about three-fifths the length of a football field, with twenty-foot wings extending at right angles on each end. In addition to the ground floor, there were three stories, accommodating two kitchens, the apothecary's shop, a servants' room, the dining room, and "twelve cells for mad people." Woven through the middle of the building like a great artery was a spacious staircase that allowed the passage of "street chairs" so attendants could carry people with fractures, dislocations, and dangerous wounds onto the wards without difficulty. Most patients were confined to the first and second floors, while those requiring surgery recovered on the third floor, where they had greater access to fresh air. In the attic was a large operating theater in which two hundred surgical students wedged themselves each week to witness operations.

For Lister—whose opportunities to grow under Erichsen had been stymied by the dwindling number of surgical beds at University College Hospital, following the deaths of Liston and Potter—it was an extraordinary chance to gain the clinical experience he so craved. Shortly after his arrival, he wrote to his father, "If the day were twice as long I should have abundant occupation for it, and such an occupation as I believe will be valuable to me for life, if I like to practise surgery." Lister's trip to Edinburgh kept being extended.

Lister quickly became Syme's right-hand man, taking on more and more responsibility at the Royal Infirmary and assisting him with complex surgeries. In a letter to his sister Mary, Lister wrote that the elder surgeon had woken him at five o'clock the previous morning to help with an emergency operation because "Mr. Syme [thought] it would amuse me." Lister went on to tell his sister that his plans to remain in Scotland for only a month had changed:

> My present opportunities are teaching me what I could not
> learn from any books, nor indeed from anybody else, while
> my experience, which our small hospital in Gower Street
> had left considerably limited, is daily receiving important
> additions. I am therefore quite satisfied that it will be well
> for me, if all goes well, to spend the winter here and even
> though my doing so should make my visit to the Continent
> exceedingly short.

A few days later, Syme invented a position for his protégé as "supernumerary clerk" because the role of house surgeon was already taken. The fact that Lister—a fully qualified surgeon in his own right and a Fellow of the Royal College of Surgeons of England—accepted a job that was more suited for a student speaks to Syme's influence over him. Equally, Syme was plainly impressed enough with Lister to have created the post for him and to have appointed him over his other students.

Syme took a keen interest in Lister's career and came to rely on him, both inside and outside the Royal Infirmary. He assigned Lister the important task of writing up reports of his clinical lectures for publication. The first appeared in the *Monthly Journal of Medical Science* and included some of Lister's own microscopic observations of a bone tumor's cellular structure. Two other papers were quick to follow: one on an operation that Syme performed on a carbuncle, and another on the use of a hot-iron cautery as a counterirritant against pain and swelling. Both of these papers included original contributions from Lister himself.

Syme became a source of inspiration. In a letter back home, Lister gushed, "If the love of surgery is a proof of a person's being adapted for it, then certainly I am fitted to be a surgeon: for thou canst hardly conceive what a high degree of enjoyment I am from day to day experiencing in this bloody and butchering department of the healing art." So enthralled was Lister by Syme that he had to justify his admiration to his father, who had sent him a letter—half playful, half in earnest—warning his son to be wary of falling too far under one man's sway: *"Nullius jurare in verba magistri"* (Swear allegiance to no master).

Although his father fretted about it, Lister defended the amount of time he spent assisting Syme: "I am pleased to be a means of aiding in the diffusion of his many original views in Surgery. . . . Had it not been for the publication of his lectures, much of his wisdom must have gone whenever he went himself." What's more, he told his father that although he agreed in theory with his warning to swear allegiance to no master, on reflection he considered Syme a very worthy "magister."

Joseph Jackson wasn't alone in taking note of his son's infatuation with the elder surgeon. Word had gotten back to London about Lister's newfound friendship with the quarrelsome Scotsman. Writing to Lister, his friend and former student George Buchanan teased, "Why! You must be in a perpetual state of bliss of the most aggravated description. . . . We saw your name in the papers as an adopted child of Syme's, reporting a case for him." Buchanan went on to add a warning of his own: "Become Syme's equal, if you will in Surgery, but pray don't catch his only too apparent egotism!"

Despite other people's concerns, Lister soared under Syme's guidance. At the Royal Infirmary, he was exposed to a far greater variety of cases than he had ever encountered in London. Like any surgeon at that time, Lister experienced failure, and patients died. But there were also deeply satisfying moments, such as the time a young man came through the doors of the Royal Infirmary after being stabbed in the neck—an injury that under normal circumstances in this period would have been fatal.

The boy had been both lucky and unlucky. On the one hand, the knife had failed to sever the carotid artery, which, had it been cut, would have ended his life instantaneously. On the other hand, blood was collecting around his windpipe, slowly cutting off his air supply. One witness remarked, "Two lives . . . depended upon the slow, progressive leakage from the wounded artery," because the assailant would undoubtedly be hanged if the young man died.

Syme and Lister wasted no time. The boy was hoisted up four flights of stairs to the attic of the Royal Infirmary, where the two surgeons began preparing for the operation. Word of what was happening quickly spread throughout the hospital, and the operating theater soon filled with surgeons and students, who jostled with one another to witness the unfolding drama. These witnesses to a potential death stood rapt in the auditorium as the patient gurgled and choked on his own blood. One spectator wrote that on every face "there was written the anxiety and dread which leavens all curiosity."

Syme looked cool and collected compared with Lister, no doubt acutely aware of the awesome responsibility facing him as he braced himself for the gore. Syme picked up the knife and traced the long red line of an incision down the young man's neck. At once, a deep pool of blood began to form around the opening. Undeterred, the senior surgeon continued to cut swiftly toward the injured artery. As Syme later wrote: "Even now I cannot, without a shudder, reflect on my position, when the slightest displacement of one hand must have instantaneously caused a fatal hemorrhage from the carotid artery, and a wrong direction of the needle by the other, to the smallest possible extent, would have given issue to an irrepressible stream from the jugular vein."

The seconds ticked by. The audience leaned forward, but all they could see were "gouts of blood spouting and welling from the wound, and the surgeon's and assistant's quick fingers at work." The patient's face grew "ghastly in its whiteness." Lister's own face, he noted, was bathed in sweat, "as if he had been running a race."

The two surgeons pressed on. Syme pushed his fingers into the open incision and with a blunt needle and a piece of silk began to tie off the injured artery. Suddenly blood erupted from the boy's neck, drenching the wooden operating table and congealing at Lister's feet. The spectators gasped, expecting death to follow quickly. But Syme continued to close the slippery artery as Lister held open the wound and sponged away the blood. After several tense minutes, both Syme and Lister backed away from the operating table so that the audience could inspect the incision. The bleeding had been halted.

A silence fell upon the theater for several seconds, before the spell was broken by the crowd erupting into riotous cheers and hurrahs for the two surgeons.

In January 1854, Lister became Syme's house surgeon, a role he had more or less been fulfilling already. In this official position, he now had twelve dressers working under him—three times more than he did at University College Hospital. This number would soon grow to twenty-three. Syme made it clear that their working relationship would be collegial and that "house surgeon" was merely a title. Syme promised not to interfere in the treatment of ordinary cases and would allow Lister the exceptional privilege of selecting his own patients from those already on the wards—something no other house surgeon could expect at any other hospital. Because Lister was not yet licensed in Scotland, however, he would only be able to assist Syme in operations at the Royal Infirmary, not lead them.

Lister quickly gained the respect and adoration of those who worked with him. The solemnity and decorum that had often characterized his behavior at UCL seemed to dissolve amid the young and sometimes rowdy group of residents in his charge. Lister even threw several lavish dinner parties for his subordinates and joined them in helping to tear down an advertisement that had been erected by a local quack doctor. The triumphant mob took the billboard and burned it in a mock ceremony on the hospital's grounds.

The dressers and clerks dubbed Syme "the Master" and Lister "the Chief"—a term of endearment that stuck with him for the rest of his life. One member of the staff in particular took a shine to the handsome surgeon: the formidable Mrs. Janet Porter, matron of the hospital and head of the nursing staff at the Royal Infirmary.

At the time of Lister's appointment, nursing was not a calling that required skill or training, nor did it command much respect. Educated, well-to-do women didn't dare enter a profession that would expose them to the intimate workings of the male body or leave them alone and unsupervised with men. Florence Nightingale—the woman who would later revolutionize nursing—had not yet fully developed the protocols of cleanliness for which she would become celebrated. Furthermore, it would be another nine years before the founding of the International Red Cross, which would be instrumental in training nurses in the latter half of the nineteenth century.

As a result of the profession's low recruitment standards, many of the nurses with whom Lister worked were a motley crew. Nightingale herself once visited the Royal Infirmary and found it to be a "lawless" place when it came to managing the nursing staff. She explained that it was the senior house surgeon's duty to have the "drunken night nurses carried in on stretchers every night." This unpleasant task would have fallen to Lister in his first year working under Syme. Indeed, there was a woman who used the hospital beds to sleep off her frequent hangovers and whom Lister had to reprimand on several occasions.

Lister's admirer Mrs. Porter was at the opposite end of the spectrum from these alcoholic loafers. She ruled the surgeons with an iron fist and behaved as if the entire burden of responsibility for managing the hospital rested on her shoulders alone. When Lister arrived at the hospital, Mrs. Porter was already firmly established there, having cared for its patients for over a decade. Her sitting room was a veritable photographic portrait gallery of the medical men who had passed through her wards. Over the years, she would come to bridge the gap between the old vanguard of nursing and the new, and she was equally adored and feared by those who knew her. The poet W. E. Henley, who was treated by Lister later in his career, wrote about the "depth and malice of her sly gray eyes" and the "broad Scots tongue that flatters, scolds, defies." Like all those who worked for Syme, she exuded an acute sense of duty. As Henley said, "Doctors love her, tease her, use her skill," but "they say 'The Chief' himself is half afraid of her."

There were many times when the new surgeon found himself in hot water with Mrs. Porter. In one instance, she caught Lister trying to break one of her ice poultices into small pieces with the ward poker. One account recalled: "[In] high dudgeon, she snatched poker and poultice from him and retreated in loud-voice remonstrance into her kitchen."

In spite of all the bluster, Mrs. Porter truly took a motherly interest in Lister's well-being. This was at no time more apparent than when he found himself crumpled in pain on the treacherous trail known as the Cat's Nick, with his former UCL classmate John Beddoe, on a blustery Sunday afternoon in 1854. The Cat's Nick cut a jagged path up the Salisbury Crags, which loom high above Edinburgh like an imposing fortress. Situated less than half a mile southeast of the city's center, the 151-foot cliffs are the glaciated remains of a carboniferous sill that began to form in a shallow sea some 340 million years ago. Lister—who was terrified of heights— had reluctantly accepted his friend's challenge to scale a precipitous face on Salisbury Crags so that they might view the magnificence of Edinburgh from an elevated position. Beddoe told Lister that all the great thinkers had done so: the novelist Sir Walter Scott, the poet Robert Burns. It had even been taken on by Charles Darwin, an enthusiastic walker who later credited his solitary rambles on Salisbury Crags for his acceptance of the geologist James Hutton's notion of deep time, a concept that would later play a crucial role in his theory of evolution. For Beddoe, it was a "feat not to be left undone."

And so the two slowly began their ascent. Step by step, the city dropped away. As they reached the halfway point, Lister started to doubt whether he could reach the top. He shouted to his friend ahead of him, "I feel giddy; would it not be foolish in me to persevere today?" Perhaps Beddoe saw the fear in his friend's eyes, or perhaps he himself was too exhausted to go any farther. He agreed that they should turn back.

As the two retraced their steps, Beddoe slipped, releasing a boulder. Lister heard a fragment come free and looked up just in time to see his friend and the rock hurtling toward him. He pressed his back against the face of the cliff just as Beddoe managed to regain his footing, but the huge rock struck Lister on the thigh. According to Lister's friend, it "whirled down the talus below with leaps and bounds, and passed harmless through the middle of a group of children who were playing hopscotch."

Beddoe quickly assessed that the situation was grave. Leaving his injured companion behind, he scrambled down the Cat's Nick and returned shortly with a litter and four men, who carried the wounded Lister back to the hospital in a solemn procession. At the gates of the Royal Infirmary stood Mrs. Porter, wringing her hands and weeping. In her thick Scottish accent, she scolded Beddoe for putting her favorite surgeon in harm's way: "Eh, Doketur Bedie! Doketur Bedie! A kent weel hoo it wad be. Ye Englishmen are aye saefulish, gaeing aboot fustlin upo' Sawbath."

Lister was laid up for several weeks, once again delaying departure from Edinburgh. Fortunately, he hadn't broken any bones, though he had severely bruised his leg. Beddoe's nerves were shaken by the thought of how close they had come to death. Years later, he reflected on how the course of history might have been changed had Lister died: "If I had killed my friend Lister that summer . . . how many would have been lost to the world and to millions of its denizens."

6.

THE FROG'S LEGS

—

**Everywhere questions arose; everything remained
without explanation; all was doubt and difficulty.
Only the great number of the dead
was an undoubted reality.**

—IGNAZ SEMMELWEIS

T**HE THUNDERING OF CANNON REVERBERATED** around the
battlefield. Bullets whizzed through the air, tearing apart flesh and
mutilating anyone who stood in their path. Limbs were ripped
off, and entrails spilled, staining the grass crimson with the blood of
those who were often too shocked by their own injuries to cry out.
Like many young men who had never seen the horrors of war firsthand, Richard James Mackenzie was woefully unprepared for what
awaited him on the battlefield. Armed with little more than a bag of

surgical instruments and some chloroform, he joined the Seventy-Second Highlanders in their fight against the Russians at the start of the Crimean War in 1854.

The thirty-three-year-old Mackenzie had taken a sabbatical from his job as Syme's assistant to volunteer as a military surgeon. Both Mackenzie and Lister worked under Syme at the same time but in different capacities; the former was more senior, having been at the Royal Infirmary for many years. During Mackenzie's time at the hospital, he had adopted many of the elder surgeon's techniques, including the famous amputation at the ankle joint. It was because of their close working relationship that many members of the faculty at the University of Edinburgh believed Mackenzie would one day succeed Syme in his clinical professorship—the most coveted of all three surgical chairs due to its permanent allotment of hospital wards at the Royal Infirmary. But when Sir George Ballingall, the professor of military surgery, announced his own retirement, Mackenzie saw an opportunity to fast-track his career. The only thing standing in the way of securing the appointment was battlefield experience.

Soon after Mackenzie departed Edinburgh, he discovered that his meager medical supplies would be of limited value. What had most concerned Mackenzie wasn't the bullets or cannonballs but the effects that the filthy battlefield conditions had on soldiers fighting in the conflict. In a letter back home, he wrote, "We had, as you know, a nasty time of it . . . not so much from the actual mortality, as from the vast amount of sickness." Malaria, dysentery, smallpox, and typhoid fever swept through army encampments, draining the strength of forces before any battles had even commenced. Mackenzie bemoaned the fact that the men had been "brought out there to rot without firing a shot, or even getting a sight of the enemy."

Their chance arrived on September 20, when the French and British forces came together to fight the Russians in a pitched battle just south of the river Alma in the Crimea. It was to be the first major engagement of the war. The Allies won the day, but not without sustaining enormous fatalities. Mackenzie's side suffered approximately twenty-five hundred casualties, while the Russians incurred over twice that number. The Battle of the Alma was a bloodbath: in addition to extracting numerous bullets and dressing a multitude of wounds for his fallen comrades, Mackenzie had to perform twenty-seven operations that day alone (including two amputations at the hip joint), all in makeshift hospital tents.

Those who survived the combat and loss of limbs were not clear of danger just yet. Shortly after the guns fell silent, there was an outbreak of Asiatic cholera. It stalked Mackenzie's battalion across water, over hills, and through valleys. It was relentless in its pursuit. Generated by the bacterium *Vibrio cholerae*, this disease is usually transmitted through water supplies contaminated by the feces of the infected. At the time of the Crimean War, the disease was making its way across Europe—and it's possible that the cholera was carried to the front line in the guts of soldiers. After an incubation period of two to five days, a victim will suffer the sudden onset of severe diarrhea and vomiting, giving rise to massive fluid loss and dehydration. Death can follow within hours, as Mackenzie noted in a letter back home: "Many were struck down at morning parade, and died in three, four, or five hours. . . . I need scarcely say, that any treatment in such cases was utterly vain." If left untreated, Asiatic cholera has a 40–60 percent mortality rate.

During the two-and-a-half-year conflict, more than eighteen thousand soldiers would die from the disease, which claimed more lives than any other that plagued the British army during the Crimean War. Among the first to succumb was Richard James Mackenzie. The promising surgeon from Edinburgh died of cholera five days after the Battle of the Alma, on September 25, 1854. Once again, death had cleared the way for another man's advancement.

. . .

Many of Mackenzie's colleagues followed him into war, but Lister's religion forbade him from engaging in violent acts, even if his role as surgeon would focus on healing the wounded. As his house surgeoncy at the Royal Infirmary drew to a close toward the end of 1854, he found himself without a job and without a plan for the future. A few months earlier, he had expressed interest to his father in applying to become a junior surgeon at the Royal Free Hospital in London. Despite his fondness for Syme, Lister missed his family. This would be the first of many attempts to return home over the next twenty-three years.

The Royal Free Hospital was founded by the surgeon William Marsden in 1828 to provide free care (as the name suggested) to those who could not afford medical treatment. While hospitals around Britain catered to the poor, patients were expected to contribute to their room and board. Additionally, inpatient admission was only granted to those who could obtain a letter from the governor or subscribers of the hospital, which was no easy task. In contrast, Marsden believed that "the only passport [to gaining admission] should be poverty and disease." His decision to erect the Royal Free was motivated by the plight of a dying girl whom he found on the steps of St. Andrew's Church one evening. Marsden tried to have her admitted to a hospital but failed because she was penniless. A few weeks later, she died.

An appointment to the Royal Free Hospital would not just bring Lister closer to home. It would also promote his career. Hospital positions were difficult to come by, especially in the capital. It would not only elevate his prestige as a surgeon, initiating a lucrative private practice, but also might lead to a university position in the future. Both Syme and his old professor William Sharpey, however, weren't so sure that this position was right for Lister. They discouraged him from applying because they feared their protégé would become entangled in one of the latest political disputes raging at the hospital.

The dispute had been all the gossip among the medical community in London. There were three surgeons at the Royal Free: William Marsden; John Gay, who had been working there for eighteen years; and Thomas Henry Wakley, whose father had founded *The Lancet*. That December, Gay had been forced to resign after he supplied information for a biography of himself that turned out to be critical of the hospital. The Committee of Governors at the Royal Free took the view that Gay had done too little to counter disparaging remarks that appeared in the book. At this point, two factions arose. Those who believed the committee was justified in pushing Gay out were pitted against those who believed a lay body shouldn't interfere in a surgeon's career. Wakley defended the committee's actions vociferously in *The Lancet*, which was not surprising, because he would benefit directly from the fallout by being promoted to Gay's position.

Sharpey wrote to Syme in Edinburgh, "The new Surgeon will be thrown much more in with young Wakley—and I fear they would not be long without a misunderstanding in which case there will be endless and distracting disputes before the public—or else Lister's retirement. I cannot imagine Lister *concurring* with Wakley in his line of proceeding." Syme had an additional concern. He worried that Lister might eclipse the quarrelsome young Wakley, which might anger Wakley's father, who still held considerable sway over the medical community in London. Sharpey wrote to Syme, "I cannot conceive of Old Wakley allowing any new man to gain reputation *at the expense of his son*." Both Sharpey and Syme relayed their concerns to Lister, who eventually allowed the deadline for an application to lapse on the advice of his two mentors.

That still left the question of what Lister would do after his house position as a surgeon ended. He considered following his original plan of traveling through Europe, and Joseph Jackson encouraged his son to do just that: "Thou art now at liberty to pursue without interruption the plan which thou hadst framed as the right one . . . to take a survey of some of the medical schools of the continent." And yet, if the allure of an appointment at the Royal Free Hospital had been almost enough to take him away from Edinburgh, a tour of Europe was not. Instead, Lister proposed to Syme that he take over Mackenzie's lectures on surgery and apply to become assistant surgeon at the Royal Infirmary.

Lister might have been overqualified to be Syme's house surgeon, but he was undoubtedly *under*qualified at that stage to be his assistant because he still wasn't licensed to practice surgery in Scotland. Lister's suggestion even came as a surprise to Syme, who immediately threw cold water on the plan. But Lister would not be deterred so easily. He took a stand. In a letter to his father, he asked, "If a man is not to take advantage of the opportunities that present themselves to him, what is he to do, or what is he good for?" In his heart, he knew he was perfectly suited to this job, even if he was punching a little above his weight. "Though at first I have sometimes been almost ready to shrink from [opportunities]," he wrote, "yet I have braced myself up with that kind of reflection that if I do not do this now how shall I be fit to do my duty as a surgeon hereafter?" For all his bravado, he still exhibited his characteristic modesty, qualifying his aspirations to his Quaker father by writing that he could not hope or expect to have a "tithe of that success" that Syme had enjoyed in his own career.

Eventually, Syme warmed to the idea of Lister as his next assistant surgeon. Lister had impressed him with both his skill as an operator and his intellectual curiosity. On April 21, Lister was elected a Fellow of the Royal College of Surgeons of Scotland, which gave him license to practice surgery in Edinburgh. Shortly after that, he moved into a fashionable residence at 3 Rutland Street, across the road from Syme's consulting rooms. His father, who continued to subsidize his living expenses, thought the rent was rather high, but he wrote to Lister that he approved of him moving into "premises that are in their character and their furnishings thoroughly respectable and suited to thy professional position." Once Lister had settled into his new lodgings, the governors of the hospital confirmed his appointment to the Royal Infirmary. In September, he collected his first fee from a patient, whom he had treated under chloroform for a dislocated ankle. Joseph Lister's career was on track.

—

AS WELL-APPOINTED as Lister's home was, it could not compete with his mentor's stately residence. Although Millbank House was only half an hour's walk from the heart of the city, it felt like a country retreat to those who visited Syme and his family there. When one entered this grand enclave, the smoke, grime, and noise of Edinburgh instantly vanished. The ivy-covered mansion overlooked gently sloping hills and well-ordered terraces, providing psychological relief from the everyday horrors Syme experienced at the Royal Infirmary. The house already had several conservatories and vineries when he bought it in the 1840s. Over the years, as Syme's wealth grew from his private practice, he added a fig house, a pineapple house, a banana house, two orchid houses, and a number of conservation walls for the growing of fruit, which could be covered in glass during the winter. It was something of a tropical paradise in an otherwise weather-beaten Scotland.

Millbank House was a lively place. Syme loved to host small dinner parties for friends, colleagues, and travelers who had come to visit the medical and scientific institutes of Edinburgh. He loathed large gatherings, preferring no more than twelve guests at a time. Lister often made the cut, and the household welcomed him.

Syme's family was large by modern standards. There was Syme's second wife, Jemima Burn, and their three children, plus his daughters Agnes and Lucy by his previous marriage. His first wife, Anne Willis, had died giving birth to their ninth child some years earlier. Seven of Syme's children from his first marriage and two from his second had died of various diseases and accidents. These bereavements served as a reminder of how impotent medicine still was in the face of death.

In addition to regular dinner invitations, Lister was asked to join the family on an excursion to visit Syme's brother-in-law at his country residence at Loch Long, on the west coast of Scotland. Lister accepted, but it wasn't just to court the good opinion of the elder Syme. His gaze had fallen upon the boss's oldest daughter, Agnes.

Agnes Syme was a tall, slender girl whose plainness was all the more apparent when she was placed in the measure against her beautiful younger sister Lucy. Agnes often pulled her long, dark hair back into a loose bun, which accentuated the delicacy of her features. In a letter back home, the besotted Lister gushed about his "precious Agnes." He told Joseph Jackson that although Miss Syme's outward appearance was "not at all showy," she was blessed with an endearing personality: "There is in her countenance an ever varying expression that artlessly displays a peculiarly guileless, honest, unaffected, and modest spirit." Most important, Lister noted, there was "no lack of sound and independent intelligence," a quality she undoubtedly inherited from her father. Lister wrote about his newfound love with few inhibitions: "On rare occasions, though to *me* not now so rare as formerly, her eye expresses the deep feeling of a *very* warm heart."

Lister's mother and father were less than enthusiastic about the prospect of this union. Agnes was a firm adherent of the Episcopal Church of Scotland, as was her family, and showed no indication that she was willing to abandon her church to join the Quakers. From early on, both of Lister's parents expressed concern. As Joseph Jackson wrote, "Thy dear mother tells me she has been persuading thee not to allow thy *other* [engagements] to absorb thee too entirely to our loss." His father warned him to do nothing that might betray that he was interested in marrying Agnes. He added (perhaps to reassure himself) that he was certain that logic would win out: "Thy judgement would at once have dismissed it as incongruous."

Despite his parents' concerns, Lister fell deeper in love. Soon, every junior at the Royal Infirmary knew that "the Chief" was pursuing the boss's daughter. After a staff dinner on a night in mid-May, one of the young men sang his own parody of a popular music hall tune titled "Villikins and His Dinah," in which Lister is mysteriously killed with a surgical knife after refusing to make an honest woman of Syme's daughter:

As Syme was a stalking the Hospital around
He seed Joseph Lister lyin' dead upon the ground
With a sharp-pointed bistoury a lyin by his side
And a billet doux a statin t'was by hemorrhage he died—

Syme tries to save the life of the fictionalized Lister by tying up the severed vessels "a dozen times o'er," but to no avail. The song ends with a jolly warning:

Now all you young surgeons take warning by 'im
And never don't by no means disobey Mister Sim;
And all young maydings what hears this sad history.
Think on Joseph, Miss Syme, & the sharp-pointed bistoury.

While the sentiment behind the parody was one of affection, the altered lyrics served as a reminder to Lister that he should tread carefully with regard to courting Agnes. Her father was not a man to be crossed.

Try as he might, though, Lister could not push Agnes from his mind. But the hard fact remained: if he was going to marry an Episcopalian, he'd have to relinquish his membership in the Quaker community. For a man who had just seven years earlier seriously contemplated giving up his medical studies to become a minister, it was a vexing decision. There weren't just religious consequences to consider; there were financial risks as well. Joseph Jackson continued to support Lister for the time being, granting him £300 per year for expenses, plus an additional £150 annual interest from his own property. However, there was no guarantee that his father would continue to pay him an allowance if he decided to stray from the flock.

Eventually, Lister asked his father outright whether he could continue to count on his financial support should he ask Agnes for her hand in marriage. Joseph Jackson put his religious concerns aside and pledged his love to his son: "I would not allow the circumstances of her not being within our society to affect my pecuniary arrangements for thee—or alter the expectations given thee some time ago." He offered his son money to buy furniture should Lister's proposal be accepted and told his son that he expected Syme would "make a settlement" on his daughter (in essence, offer a dowry) and that he would negotiate this with Syme directly.

His father assured him that neither he nor his mother wished Lister to "attend the worship of 'Friends' *for the sake of our* feelings." He suggested that his son voluntarily resign his membership in the Society of Friends, rather than be formally disowned as the Rules of Discipline would demand if he married someone of a different faith. Joseph Jackson felt this was best all around and would leave the door open if Lister ever decided to return to the Quaker community.

With his mind at rest, Lister proposed to Agnes and was accepted. Agnes and her mother set the wedding date for the following spring. Lister, eager to begin his life with his new bride, complained to his father about the delay. If it were up to him, the two would be married at once. Joseph Jackson—no doubt amused by his son's eagerness to begin enjoying the benefits of domesticity—assured him: "My preference like thine would be for the earlier, but thou wilt see that there are *reasons* why the fixing it should be left to the *ladies* [*sic*] discretion."

The wedding gifts began rolling in: a black marble clock from the Pims in Ireland; a beautiful dessert service from his brother Arthur. Lister, who had only just moved, now had to find a home that was more suited for married life. With Agnes's considerable dowry, along with money from Joseph Jackson given to them as a wedding gift, the couple could afford a more stately residence. Lister settled on 11 Rutland Street, just a few doors down from his old lodgings. This granite-faced Georgian house had nine rooms spread out over three floors, including a study just off the entrance hall, which Lister intended to convert into a consulting room for his future patients. In a letter to his mother, he also described a room on the second floor that had once been a nursery as it was "well provided with a sink with taps for hot & cold water."

On April 23, 1856, the couple were married in Syme's drawing room at Millbank House. Agnes's sister Lucy later recalled that this was done "out of consideration for any Quaker relation" who would have been uncomfortable attending a church service. The Scottish physician and essayist John Brown toasted the happy couple after the reception. Their future was bright, not least because Lister's star was rising within Edinburgh. During his speech, Brown made a prescient assertion: "Lister is one who, I believe, will go to the very top of his profession."

When Lister returned to work at the Royal Infirmary, he continued to face the same problems that had presented themselves at University College Hospital in London. Patients were dying from gangrene, erysipelas, septicemia, and pyemia. Frustrated by what most hospital surgeons accepted as an inevitability, Lister began taking samples of tissue from his patients to study under the lens of his microscope so he could better understand what was happening at a cellular level.

Like many of his colleagues, Lister recognized that excessive inflammation often preceded the onset of a septic condition. Once this occurred, a patient would develop a fever. The underlying factor linking the two seemed to be heat. Inflammation was localized heat, whereas the fever was systemic heat. In the 1850s, however, preventing either was difficult because wounds rarely healed cleanly, to the extent that many doctors considered "laudable pus" essential to the healing process. Moreover, there was a debate within the medical community as to whether inflammation was in fact "normal" or a pathogenic process that needed to be countered.

Lister was determined to better understand the mechanisms behind inflammation. What was the connection between inflammation and hospital gangrene? Why did some inflamed wounds become septic while others didn't? In a letter to his father, he wrote that he "felt that the early stages of [inflammation] had not been traced as they might be, so as to see the transition from the state of healthy increased redness to inflammation."

Controlling inflammation was a daily struggle for the hospital surgeon. Contemporaries believed that a wound could heal in one of two ways. The ideal situation was if a wound healed by "first intention," a term used by surgeons to denote the reuniting of the two sides with minimal inflammation and suppuration (formation of pus). Put simply, the wound healed cleanly, or "sweetly," to use a term of the period. Alternatively, a wound might heal by "second intention" through the development of new granulations or scar tissue—a prolonged process that was frequently accompanied by both inflammation and suppuration. Wounds that healed by second intention were more likely to become infected, or "sour."

The ways in which surgeons managed wounds were numerous and demonstrate just how much they struggled to understand and control inflammation, suppuration, and fever. Complicating matters was the fact that the development of septic infections seemed arbitrary and unpredictable at times. Some wounds healed beautifully with little medical assistance, while others proved fatal despite being carefully managed through frequent dressing changes and debridement (the removal of dead tissue). One phenomenon many surgeons noticed was that simple fractures resulting in no break of the skin often healed without incident. This reinforced the idea that something had entered the wound from outside, which in turn gave rise to the popular "occlusion method" that sought to exclude air from a wound.

The occlusion method could be achieved in multiple ways according to the preference of the surgeon handling the case. The first was to cover the wound entirely with a dry dressing, such as goldbeater's skin made from the outer membrane of a calf's intestine, or an adhesive plaster. If the wound healed by first intention, this method was successful. But if suppuration occurred, the putrefactive poison (or bacteria, as we know it today)—unable to escape from underneath the dressing's constraints—would be redirected into the patient's bloodstream, and septicemia would occur. To counter this effect, some surgeons continually reopened the dressing to clean out the discharge in a method called "occlusion with repeated opening." Robert Liston, in fact, denounced this practice in the 1840s, noting that "the patient is kept in a state of constant excitement, and often, worn out by suffering, discharge, and hectic fever, falls a victim to the practice."

Many surgeons were against the occlusion method because it trapped heat inside the wound, which was counterintuitive when it came to controlling inflammation. They also believed that the injured site should not be covered up entirely, because the bandages would become "loaded with putrid exhalations, and a profusion of bloody, ill-digested, foetid matter," and this, in turn, would make the wound go sour. Syme preferred to stitch up the wound, leaving a small opening for drainage. Afterward, he wrapped everything but the portal with a broad piece of dry lint. This was left undisturbed for about four days, at which time the lint was removed and changed every second day until the wound had healed.

Some surgeons preferred "water dressings," or wet bandages, which they believed counteracted the heat of inflammation by keeping the wound cool. Others tried irrigating the wound directly, and even immersed the whole patient in water that constantly had to be changed. Although this method proved the most successful because it inadvertently removed discharge as soon as it was formed, it was expensive and awkward to enact, and there was much disagreement as to whether the water should be hot, tepid, or cold.

The biggest problem was that while a majority of surgeons tried to prevent wound infections, there was no consensus as to *why* they happened in the first place. Some believed that the cause was some kind of poison in the air, but it was anybody's guess what the nature of that poison actually was. Others thought that wound infection could arise de novo through the process of spontaneous generation, especially if a patient was already in a weakened state.

Nearly everyone in the medical community recognized that hospital settings were a contributing factor to the rise of infection rates in recent years. More and different types of patients were admitted to hospitals as they grew in size during the nineteenth century. This was especially true after the advent of anesthesia in 1846, which gave surgeons more confidence to take on operations that they would not necessarily have dared undertake before that innovation. With so many patients on the wards, keeping the hospitals clean became increasingly difficult. The author of an important textbook, *Year-Book of Medicine, Surgery, and Their Allied Sciences*, felt the need to advise readers, "The bandages and instruments which have been employed for gangrenous wounds ought not, if possible, to be employed a second time; nor should bandages, linen, or clothing, be prepared or kept in rooms where infected patients are lying. Frequent change of the bedding, blankets, and linen, is also of the greatest utility where these diseases have already broken out."

The level of hygiene that we expect in hospitals today simply did not exist, and certainly was not present at the Royal Infirmary when Lister began his work there. Finding some route to an understanding of the nature of inflammation and infection had become more critical than ever.

—

DURING THE FIRST YEAR of their marriage, Agnes grew accustomed to the sight of frogs in the marital home. Her husband's obsession with the amphibians began on their honeymoon. Before heading off on a four-month tour of Europe, the newlyweds had stopped at an uncle's house in Kinross, just a day's travel from Edinburgh by horse and carriage. Lister brought his microscope with him and, having caught some frogs just outside the uncle's property, rigged up a laboratory in order to begin a series of experiments that he hoped would help him better understand the process of inflammation—a subject that would consume him for the rest of his life. Unfortunately for Lister (though happily for the frogs), they managed to escape on this occasion, causing uproar in the house as the servants scurried around trying to catch them. After the couple returned from their travels, Lister resumed his experiments, this time in his own laboratory on the ground floor of his Rutland Street home. He worked

tirelessly with his diligent wife by his side. Agnes often took dicta-
tion, recording his notes in meticulous handwriting in his casebooks.
Indeed, there seemed to be little time for anything but study.

Until this time, Lister had mostly examined dead tissue under
the microscope. These samples were often taken from patients he cared
for at the Royal Infirmary or, in some cases, even sourced from his
own body. But what he really needed was *living* tissue in order to
understand exactly how blood vessels reacted under different circumstances. This was a crucial step in his understanding of wound care
and the causes of postoperative infections. Once more, he turned his
attention to live frogs, this time visiting Duddingston Loch to the east
of the city center to procure a batch for research into the subject. It
was then that he began to unravel the mystery that had troubled his
profession for centuries.

Lister's investigations into inflammation were a continuation of
earlier work conducted by his UCL professor Wharton Jones, who
made some microscopic observations on peripheral blood vessels by
using the translucent tissues of bat wings and webs from the feet of
frogs. Like his old professor, Lister recognized that the slowing of
blood through the capillaries seemed to precede the onset of infection.
What he wanted to understand was how inflammation affected
blood vessels and blood flow in healthy limbs. In his home lab, he
devised a series of experiments in which he inflicted controlled and
graduated injuries on a frog's webs, measuring the diameter of blood
vessels with an ocular micrometer on each occasion. To do this, he
placed various irritants on the webs, beginning with warm water
made incrementally hotter with each application until it finally reached
the boiling point. Next, Lister tested the effects of chloroform, mus-
tard, croton oil, and acetic acid on the webs.

Crucial to his experiments was pinpointing the role that the
central nervous system played in inflammation. To understand
this better, Lister vivisected a large frog and proceeded to remove its

entire brain without injuring the spinal cord. (The act of cutting into live animals for the purposes of scientific investigation had a long history in Britain. In 1664, Robert Hooke—a founding member of the Royal Society and pioneer of the microscope—strapped a stray dog to his laboratory table and proceeded to slice the terrified animal's chest away so he could peer inside the thoracic cavity and better understand the mechanisms involved in breathing. What Hooke hadn't realized before he began his experiment was that lungs were not muscles, and that by removing the animal's chest and disabling the diaphragm, he had destroyed the dog's ability to breathe on its own. To keep the animal alive, Hooke pushed a hollow cane down the dog's throat and into its windpipe. He then pumped air into the animal's lungs with bellows for over an hour, carefully studying the way in which the organs expanded and contracted with each artificial breath. All the while, the dog stared at him in horror, unable to whimper or howl in agony. Like Hooke, Lister saw vivisection as a necessary evil of his profession, one invaluable to his own research and to saving the lives of his patients.)

After he had removed the frog's brain, he observed that "the arteries, which had previously been pretty full size and transmitting rapid streams of blood, were found completely contracted, so that the webs appeared bloodless except in the veins." Over the next several hours, Lister continued to manipulate the spinal cord, even at times removing bits of it, until the frog died: "The blood had ceased to move in consequence of the feebleness of the heart." He deduced that arteries in frogs without brains or spinal cords did not dilate.

Lister decided to present his findings to the Royal College of Surgeons in Edinburgh. When the time came to deliver his speech, however, he still hadn't concluded his experiments to his own satisfaction. With the clock ticking, his father—who was visiting the young couple in Scotland—noted that his son had only completed half of his speech by the night before and that "one third had to be spoken *extempore*" on the day of delivery. But for all his unpreparedness, the paper was given without a hitch, and a version of it was published in the *Philosophical Transactions of the Royal Society*.

In the paper, Lister contended that "a certain amount of inflammation as caused by direct irritation is essential to primary union." In other words, inflammation resulting from an incision or a fracture was to be expected when a wound was sustained and was indeed very much a part of the body's natural healing process. Inflammation of a wound did not necessarily presage sepsis. In opposition to Wharton Jones, Lister argued that the vascular tone of a frog's leg was under the control of the spinal cord and medulla oblongata, and thus inflammation could be directly affected by the central nervous system. Put plainly, Lister believed that there were two kinds of inflammations: local and nervous.

In his concluding remarks, Lister chronicled his experimental observations of the frogs, relating them to clinical situations such as trauma caused to skin by boiling water or surgical incisions. These early studies were crucial to Lister's future clinical work on the healing of wounds and the effects of infection on tissues. He was ultimately incorrect in believing that there were two types of inflammations, but through his groundbreaking work he secured a better grasp of the effects that inflammation had on the loss of vitality in tissues. This was of paramount importance in helping him understand why sepsis conditions were likely to develop in damaged tissue.

Even after his lecture at the Royal College of Surgeons, and when he wasn't lecturing or treating patients at the Royal Infirmary, he continued his intensive experimentation on frogs, with Agnes's help. This prompted Joseph Jackson to write to him: "I am ready to ask what new points . . . render requisite still further experiments with the poor frogs." It would not be the last time Lister's thoroughness and attention to detail would be a hindrance to the timely publication of important research. Nevertheless, during the first three years of his marriage, he managed to publish fifteen papers, nine of which appeared in 1858 alone. All of them were based on his original findings, and many of them detailed the results of his physiological investigations into the origin and mechanism of inflammation, which gave him a solid foundation on which to build his seminal work.

7.

CLEANLINESS AND COLD WATER

—

The surgeon is like the husbandman, who having sown
his field, waits with resignation for what the harvest
may bring, and reaps it, fully conscious of his own
impotence against the elemental powers, which may
pour down on him rain, hurricane and hail storm.

—RICHARD VON VOLKMANN

IN JULY 1859, JAMES LAWRIE—the fifty-nine-year-old Regius Professor of Clinical Surgery at the University of Glasgow—suffered a paralytic stroke that robbed him of the ability to move or speak. He was well known at the university and had even taught the famous medical missionary and explorer David Livingstone. Lawrie's position, coveted by many within the surgical community, was suddenly in play.

Lister immediately wrote to his father with the news: "Dr. Lawrie . . . is in such a state of health as cannot permit him to hold his office much longer." He expressed interest in applying for the position himself. With such a prestigious title, he would be able to grow his own lucrative private practice in Glasgow, something he had not been able to do in Edinburgh. Moreover, Lister assumed that he would be appointed surgeon to the city's hospital through the influence of his friends who were part of the medical faculty there. Most important, as he told his father, he felt confident that if he was to secure the position, it would give him "greater claim to any London appointment" that might arise in the future.

But there was a downside. If Lister moved to Glasgow, it would spell an end to his six-year partnership with his friend, colleague, and father-in-law. He lamented to Joseph Jackson, "I should very much regret leaving Edinburgh, and particularly Mr. Syme, for whom, as thee know, I have a very deep regard." Lister also fretted about what it might mean for his old mentor and the surgical practice they had cultivated over the past few years: "Mr. Syme . . . would evidently be more agreeable that I should stay here and help him at the hospital . . . for there is no one else in this town who is on the same sort of footing with him as myself in surgical matters." Despite this, the thirty-two-year-old surgeon could not ignore the opportunities that would await him were he to take up a professorship in Glasgow. He set aside his attachment to Syme and the Royal Infirmary and put his name forward for the post.

Seven other highly skilled candidates also applied for the position: five from Glasgow, two from Edinburgh. Complicating matters was the fact that all appointments for Regius Professorships in Britain were in the hands of a minister of the Crown, who was unlikely to know much about the specific requirements of any given post or which candidates might be best qualified to fill it. Syme graciously recommended his son-in-law, noting in characteristically terse language that Lister had a "strict regard for accuracy, extremely correct powers of observation, and a remarkably sound judgment, united to uncommon manual dexterity and a practical turn of mind."

Time elapsed, but still there was no word about the position. Then, in December, Lister received a private letter from a confidant who informed him that he would be offered the Regius Professorship. But his elation was soon dampened when *The Glasgow Herald* announced in January that the matter had not yet been settled. The article drew attention to an open letter that had been circulated throughout the medical community by the city's two MPs, who asked local doctors to "inform us which candidate is, in your opinion, the best qualified for the appointment, by placing a cross opposite to his name." There was an outcry from those concerned about corruption and patronage. If a candidate was handpicked by Glaswegian doctors, then surely there would be a bias against outsiders like Lister.

The protest grew, with William Sharpey, John Eric Erichsen, and James Syme all writing letters in support of Lister's candidacy. Ten days after the editorial appeared, Lister was asked officially by the home secretary to fill Lawrie's position. The following day, a jubilant son wrote to his father, "At last the welcome news has arrived . . . that Her Majesty has approved of my appointment." Lister described feeling "intoxicated with [a] gladness" that had been "doubled or trebled, I doubt not, by the long period of suspense that preceded it." As a happy consequence, he also believed that the decision had cleared Glasgow of the charge of narrow-mindedness and clannishness universally made against it. In this new city, Lister believed he and Agnes would make themselves at home.

Glasgow was only forty miles from Edinburgh. An ancient university was at the heart of both cities, but the intellectual atmosphere in Glasgow was very different from the one that Lister had grown accustomed to in Edinburgh while working alongside Syme. The Glaswegian medical community was more authoritarian than speculative, more conservative than maverick. It did not welcome innovation readily. Lister would struggle to find his place amid the more traditionally minded stalwarts at the university.

When Lister arrived for his induction ceremony, the room was crowded with distinguished men from the institution, the same people who would soon be his colleagues. They had congregated in droves to hear the new professor of clinical surgery give his first speech. Lister was anxious. A day earlier, he had been told that he would have to deliver his thesis in Latin, an antiquated tradition that stemmed from the belief that medical men should be able to exhibit their breadth of learning. One contemporary wrote, "We ought to be men and gentlemen first before we are doctors or men of science."

Into the late hours the night before, Lister struggled to prepare his important speech. Now, as he stood before the audience, he nervously clutched at a Latin dictionary that he had brought along at Agnes's suggestion. To compound his angst, he also worried that his stutter would return, as it sometimes did when he was under intense pressure. But as he began to speak, he fell into a rhythm. The Latin rolled off his tongue with surprising ease. Just as he was about to launch into further passages of his thesis, the principal of the university rose out of his seat and interrupted him. He indicated that Lister could stop because he had already satisfied the requirements with the first few paragraphs of his paper. He had passed his first test.

The University of Glasgow's conservative leanings notwithstanding, changes were under way. Recent appointments to the faculty attracted newcomers and helped offset the institution's somewhat flagging reputation. In 1846, William Thomson (known as Lord Kelvin, who later formulated the first and second laws of thermodynamics) joined the faculty as professor of natural philosophy, bringing with him an emphasis on laboratory and experimental work in the classroom. Two years later, Allen Thomson became professor of anatomy. His lectures on microscopic anatomy were a novel addition to the university's otherwise stale curriculum. As a result of these changes, the university began to see a steady rise in its intake of medical students. When Lister joined the faculty, there were 311 students registered, nearly three times the number enrolled just twenty years earlier. Of these, over half had signed up for Lister's new course on systematic surgery, making it the largest of its kind in Britain.

The university was not equipped for this sudden influx of students. While Edinburgh had allocated hundreds of pounds for renovation of its classrooms and teaching apparatus, Glasgow offered virtually nothing in the way of financial investment. Lister—whose practical teaching methods required the use of anatomical specimens, models, and drawings—found the lecture theater assigned to him to be inadequate. He decided to invest his own money in renovating the space, and the measures he undertook included the building of a "retiring room" attached to the theater where he could store his unusual specimen collection. The desks and chairs were also replaced, and the entire room was cleaned and eventually repainted. Agnes helped with the redecorating. Writing to Lister's mother, Isabella, in May, she noted, "How nice it looks . . . the green baize on the three doors and the diagram-frame setting off the oak colouring, and the bright little brass handles on the doors setting them off; and the very handsome slate on the frame on one side and the skeleton nicely mounted on the other. Some plates are hung on a diagram-frame and some preparations are on the nice oak-table." The refurbishments had an instantaneous effect on Lister's incoming students, who removed their hats upon entering the lecture theater and waited in reverent silence after taking their seats. The fresh surroundings signaled to them that they could expect an equally fresh approach to their education.

Despite his lingering concerns about speaking in front of a large crowd, Lister's first lecture there was an unqualified success. He opened with a quotation from the sixteenth-century surgeon Ambroise Paré, who famously said, "I dressed him, God cured him," before moving on to a discussion about the importance of anatomy and physiology in surgery. Lister's discourse was both informative and entertaining. His nephew said that the students "laughed, too, in the right places" as the normally reserved Quaker made a "quiet gentlemanly hit at homeopathy," which he had been condemning since his student days at UCL.

One of the principal topics of his talk was on making serviceable stumps when amputating limbs so that amputees could regain as much function as possible and wouldn't become burdens on their families or society. Again, he had the room bursting into laughter when he told them a story about a stoic youth from Scotland who was able to dance the Highland fling after Lister had removed both of the man's legs. After the lecture, Lister wrote to his mother, "I now feel, that with the same gracious help I can do anything. . . . It was curious how entirely absent any shade of anxiety was during the whole proceedings."

The students immediately warmed to their new professor, who in turn became more comfortable in his role as their teacher. They were even grateful for his tendency to stutter, which forced him to speak slowly and enabled them to take notes more easily. One of his graduates later wrote that Lister was in fact worshipped by his students. Back in Edinburgh, Syme also heard of his protégé's progress. He wrote to his son-in-law, "The game may be considered in your own hands," adding, almost as an afterthought, "Wishing you all comfort in playing it out."

• • •

Shortly after his appointment to the university, Lister was elected a Fellow of the Royal Society—an extraordinary honor at this early stage of his career. It was a distinction his father had also had bestowed upon him, in recognition of his development of the first achromatic lens. Joseph Jackson was thrilled by the news of his son's joining him as a society member. Lister joined a long line of illustrious members, whose names included Robert Boyle, Sir Isaac Newton, and Charles Darwin. The vote was a tribute to the originality of his research into inflammation and coagulation of the blood, which he presented in a series of papers to the Royal Society in 1860.

Lister was deeply ensconced in this work at the university when he applied for a position as a surgeon at Glasgow's Royal Infirmary. He believed a hospital post was crucial to his role as a teacher, as it would allow him to demonstrate his theories and methods to students on real living patients. Before taking up his professorship, he had been told by friends in the medical faculty that his appointment to the Royal Infirmary would be all but guaranteed once he had settled into his academic role. Indeed, Lister had disclosed this expectation when he had first written to his father about Lawrie's retirement and the vacancy at the university. It therefore came as a great surprise to Lister when his application was rejected.

Lister put his case before David Smith, a boot- and shoemaker who was also the chairman of the hospital's board. One could buy one's way onto the board by making a large donation, so it was not uncommon for a hospital to be managed by people like Smith who had no medical background. The Royal Infirmary's board had twenty-five directors. Two were medical professors at the university, but the rest were a mishmash of religious officials, politicians, and other representatives of public bodies; they were hardly scientific visionaries. It was inevitable that Lister—a man who was trying to reform surgical practice from within and at a fundamental level—would come up against someone like Smith, who thought hospitals existed for only one reason: to treat patients. In the eyes of Lister and progressive contemporaries such as James Syme, a hospital was much more than this: it was a place where students could learn from real-life cases.

Lister explained to Smith that it was important as professor of clinical surgery to be able to perform demonstrations for students on the wards of the hospital so that they could unite theory with practice. He himself was a product of this type of education. Smith thought this idea preposterous. "Stop, stop, Mr. Lister, that's a real Edinburgh idea," he told the frustrated surgeon. "Our institution is a curative one. It is not an educational one." A majority of the hospital's directors agreed with Smith and voted against Lister's appointment in 1860.

There was truth in Smith's assertion that the primary role of Glasgow's Royal Infirmary was curative. The city's population had quadrupled between 1800 and 1850 and would again between 1850 and 1925. There had been an inpouring of dispossessed Highlanders in the 1820s and thousands fleeing Ireland's potato famine in the 1840s. By the time of Lister's arrival, Glasgow was one of the largest cities in the world and was known as "the Second City of the Empire" after London. As the only major hospital in a city with a population of 400,000 people, the Royal Infirmary struggled to keep pace with the growing medical demands placed on it.

As in London and Edinburgh, crime was endemic and disease rampant. Yet Glasgow was worse than most cities in Britain at this time. On his visit to the city, the German philosopher and journalist Friedrich Engels observed, "I have seen human degradation in some of its worst phases, both in England and abroad, but I can advisedly say, that I did not believe, until I visited the wynds of Glasgow, that so large an amount of filth, crime, misery, and disease existed on one spot in any civilized country." It was a place, he said, that "no person of common humanity to animals would stable his horse in."

Glasgow was expanding its heavy manufacturing, particularly shipbuilding, engineering, locomotive construction, metalworking, and oil, and as a consequence, terrible injuries featured frequently at the hospital. There was thirty-five-year-old William Duff, who severely scalded his face and upper torso while lighting a candle over a manhole at the new Oil Works in Keith Place. There was also eighteen-year-old Joseph Neille, who was working at a local munitions factory when he placed a tin flask that he had thought contained tea onto the fire. Only after it was too late did he realize the flask was actually filled with two pounds of gunpowder. And the hospital often dealt with fractured skulls, severed hands, and fatal falls.

Given the increase in industrial accidents and the ongoing outbreaks of disease, it is understandable why David Smith thought the Royal Infirmary's primary duty was to its patients, not to its medical students and their professors. Still, Smith's view that the presence of someone like Lister would be obstructive, due to his using the wards as a teaching environment, was by no means universally held. Decades earlier, many urban hospitals outside Glasgow had recognized the benefits of forging coalitions with universities so that they could attract the best and brightest practitioners in medicine.

Most of the medical positions at the larger hospitals in Britain in 1860 were voluntary, and although there was prestige in holding them, physicians and surgeons were not paid a salary. The bulk of a surgeon's income came from two sources: private practice and fee-paying students. And with the development of clinical teaching in the hospitals of Paris and elsewhere, British students had come to expect the same rigor from their homegrown education. Hospital administrators knew that if they allowed their medical staff to teach on the wards, they could attract some of the more renowned physicians and surgeons, who would otherwise have little incentive to lend their time and expertise to an institution offering no pay. Glasgow's Royal Infirmary evidently did not share this view at the time that Lister applied for a surgical position at the hospital. This was made all the more absurd by the fact that the hospital was close to the university, which would have made a mutually beneficial alliance between the two simple to expedite.

Months passed and Lister still hadn't been given official charge of patients at the city's hospital. His students were dismayed by the delay as well, because it meant that they too could not benefit from any clinical instruction from him on the wards. They had been so taken with his lectures that they made him honorary president of their medical society. At the end of the winter course, the class went a step further to show their appreciation for their much-admired instructor. They signed a declaration in which they shared their wish that his appointment to the Royal Infirmary was imminent: "Permit us to express our hope for the sake both of the rising Profession and of the Institution itself, that in the approaching appointment of a surgeon to the Royal Infirmary your application may meet with that success which your ability and position demand." The document was signed by no fewer than 161 students.

In fact, it was nearly two years *after* Lister began teaching at the university that he was put in charge of patients at the Glasgow Royal Infirmary. Even after the motion was passed, there were continued protests from some of the hospital's managers, who expressed concern over Lister's growing reputation as a progressive. Still, Lister had won this battle, if not yet the war.

When Lister stepped onto the hospital's wards in 1861, a new surgical wing had just been constructed. Originally, the hospital contained 136 beds, but with this addition there were now 572 beds, making it twice as large as Edinburgh's Royal Infirmary and four times as large as the London hospital in which Lister trained as a student. Each surgeon was given charge of one female and two male wards, the latter of which were divided between the treatment of acute and chronic conditions. Despite having been built months earlier, the surgical wing soon proved to be one of the most insanitary places in which Lister had ever worked. As one of his colleagues noted, "Its newness had not saved it from invasion by the prevailing diseases of infected wounds."

The all-too-familiar enemies of secondary hemorrhage, septicemia, pyemia, hospital gangrene, tetanus, and erysipelas were never absent from the wards. Infective suppuration in wounds came to be expected. Lister's male acute ward was located on the ground floor, which was adjacent to the graveyard (overflowing with rotting corpses from the last cholera epidemic) and separated from it only by a thin wall. He complained of the "uppermost tier of a multitude of coffins" reaching to within a few inches of the surface of the ground and said that it was "to the disappointment of all concerned [that] this noble structure proved extremely unhealthy." There were also few provisions for the washing of hands and instruments throughout the hospital. As Lister's house surgeon reflected, "When almost every wound was foul with suppuration, it seemed natural at the time to postpone the complete cleansing of hands and instruments, until the programme of dressings and probings had been finished." Everything was veneered with grime.

Like most hospitals in the 1860s, the Royal Infirmary attracted patients who were too poor to pay for private care. Some were uneducated and illiterate. Many doctors and surgeons viewed them as socially inferior and treated them with a clinical detachment that was often dehumanizing. Lister, true to his Quaker roots, exhibited an unusual level of compassion for those on his wards. He refused to use the word "case" when referring to specific patients, choosing instead to call them "this poor man" or "this good woman." He also recommended to his students that they use "technical words" so that "nothing was said or suggested that could in any way cause them anxiety or alarm"—something that would undoubtedly be viewed as unethical today but was born purely of compassion when Lister suggested it. One of his students later recounted a time when Lister admonished an instrument clerk who had brought an uncovered tray full of knives into the operating theater. The seasoned surgeon quickly threw a towel over the tray and said in slow, sorrowful tones, "How can you have such cruel disregard for this poor woman's feelings? Is it not enough for her to be passing through this ordeal without adding unnecessarily to her sufferings by displaying this array of naked steel?"

Lister understood that being in a hospital could be a terrifying experience and followed his own golden rule: "Every patient, even the most degraded, should be treated with the same care and regard as though he were the Prince of Wales himself." He went above and beyond the call of duty when it came to putting at ease the children who were admitted to his wards. Lister's house surgeon Douglas Guthrie related a touching story later in life about a little girl who came into the hospital suffering from an abscess of the knee. After Lister treated and dressed her wound, the girl held up her doll to him. He gently took the toy from her and noticed that it was missing its tiny leg. The girl fumbled around under her pillow and— much to Lister's amusement—produced the severed limb. He shook his head ominously as he inspected his newest patient. Lister turned to Guthrie and asked for a needle and cotton. Carefully, he stitched the limb back onto the doll and with quiet delight handed it back to the little girl. Guthrie said that her "large brown eyes spoke endless gratitude, but neither uttered a word." Surgeon and child seemed to understand each other perfectly.

When pain was an unavoidable part of treatment, it was often difficult to win the trust of those who didn't fully comprehend the procedures to which they were subjected. Lister certainly had his fair share of troublesome patients, and yet this never seemed to perturb him. In one instance, a forty-year-old mill worker named in the records as "Elizabeth M'K" came into the Glasgow Royal Infirmary with an injury to her hand. Lister operated and in the coming weeks attempted to bend her fingers back in order to restore flexibility to the muscles and tendons. Unfortunately, the woman mistook his efforts for attempts to break her fingers and fled the hospital in a panic. She returned five months later, her hand all but paralyzed because she had kept it in a splint the entire time. Displaying seemingly infinite patience, Lister resumed the therapy, and the patient eventually regained some movement.

Lister personally accompanied the more serious cases back to the ward after an operation and insisted on helping to transfer the patient from the stretcher to the bed. To ensure the patient's comfort, he would arrange an assortment of small pillows and hot-water bottles, warning his attendees that the latter should be covered with flannel so the anesthetized person would not inadvertently burn him- or herself during recovery. He even helped dress the sick after surgery. One of Lister's house surgeons described how "with almost womanly care he would replace the bedclothes" of the patient, "putting them all trim and square." To those who were awake, he would first ask, "Now are you quite comfortable?" before moving on to the next bed.

Even in his private practice, he exhibited an acute empathy with patients that extended to their pockets. Consequently, Lister objected to issuing bills to those whom he treated and lectured his students that they should "not charge for [their] services as a merchant does for his goods." Reflecting the ideals of his faith, Lister believed that the greatest reward for a surgeon was the knowledge that he had performed an act of beneficence for the sick. "Shall we charge for the blood which is drawn, or the pain which we cause?" he asked his students.

When he wasn't immersed in his work at the hospital, Lister began experimenting in his home laboratory again, publishing various findings on the coagulation of the blood and inflammation. He discovered that blood remained partially fluid for several hours in a vulcanized India-rubber tube but clotted promptly if placed in an ordinary cup. He concluded that blood coagulation is caused by "the influence exerted upon it by ordinary matter, the contact of which for a very brief period effects a change in the blood, inducing a mutual reaction between its solid and fluid constituents, in which the corpuscles impart to the liquor sanguinis a disposition to coagulate." He also turned his attention to observing suppurative tissues under the microscope, including the eyeball of a rabbit, the jugular vein of a large pony, and a fresh batch of tissues excised from his own patients.

Lister designed and patented several surgical instruments, showing himself to be an innovator in operative methods as well as in wound management. These included a needle for stitching wounds, a small hook that could remove objects from the ear, and a screw tourniquet for compressing the abdominal aorta—the largest blood vessel in the human body. His best-known surgical tool was the sinus forceps. With ring handles like those of scissors, the slender six-inch blades could pick fluff out of the smallest hole.

These instruments, though useful, did little to improve mortality rates at the hospital. People continued to die in alarming numbers when hospitalism broke out on the wards. In August 1863, Lister performed surgery on the wrist of a twenty-year-old laborer named Neil Campbell. Lister had developed a method for removing diseased bone from the wrist without resorting to amputating the hand. A few months later the boy returned, his wrist once again carious. Lister repeated the operation, this time removing more of the diseased bone. While the surgery was a success, Campbell's recovery was not. Shortly afterward, he developed pyemia and died. Lister grew increasingly frustrated by his inability to prevent and manage septic conditions in his patients. His case notes catalogue the questions plaguing him: "11 P.M. Query. How does the poisonous matter get from the wound into the veins? Is it that the clot in the orifices of the cut veins suppurates, or is poisonous matter absorbed by minute veins & carried into the venous trunks?"

DESPITE HIS PROFESSIONAL DILIGENCE, Joseph Lister's personal life was troubling him. On a dreary day in March 1864, Agnes embarked on a journey to Upton to visit her in-laws. Lister's mother, Isabella, was once again very ill. She was suffering from one of the many skin conditions that preoccupied her son: erysipelas. Her daughters lived nearby, but they had families of their own and couldn't provide the level of care she needed. Although Lister had hinted, in a letter to his father during the first year of their marriage, that Agnes might be pregnant, a child had not appeared and never would. The task of caregiver fell to the childless couple.

In the meantime, a professorship at the University of Edinburgh opened up in June of that year. His good standing with his devoted students aside, Lister's relationship with the directors of his current hospital remained tense. Moreover, his hectic schedule meant he had very little time to conduct personal research. In addition to his daily visits to the Royal Infirmary, he had to deliver a lecture each day—no small task for a man as meticulous with his lesson planning as Lister was. And then there was his absence from Syme. Lister missed his time working alongside a like-minded intellectual who was never satisfied with the status quo, unlike so many of his colleagues in Glasgow. Lister also saw this Edinburgh post as an opportunity yet again to find a route back to London. As his nephew later wrote, "Lister always looked upon himself as possibly only a bird of passage in Scotland . . . and he thought, if ever a move south were contemplated, Edinburgh would be a better stepping-off place than Glasgow."

Once again, Lister faced a bitter setback. Only after he had received news of his rejection and the appointment of his opponent, James Spence, did Syme reason that Lister was better off in Glasgow. His father-in-law believed that Lister's Edinburgh candidacy, though unsuccessful, would still serve to increase his reputation in the surgical community.

With the cloud of professional defeat hanging over him, Lister received word soon after that his mother's condition had rapidly deteriorated. The situation was critical, so he packed his bags and traveled down to Upton to be at her side. On September 3, 1864, Isabella Lister lost her battle with erysipelas, the same disease that continued to haunt Lister on the wards of his own hospital.

—

TO FILL THE VOID left by his wife's death, Joseph Jackson began communicating ever more frequently with his children. "The thought that thou wilt allow me to look for letters from thee weekly, & the letters when they come, are alike gratifying to thy poor father," he wrote to his son. Lister pledged to write to his father every week— a promise he faithfully fulfilled. It was in one of these many letters that Joseph Jackson reminded his son of his advancing years. Lister reflected on this: "As thee say, I have now arrived at middle life. . . . It seems strange to think that I am half as old as a man of 70! and yet I suppose the remaining half, if passed at all in this world, will go much quicker than that which is gone. Not that it matters how quickly, if it takes us to the right goal at last."

It was during this time that Lister attempted to improve hygiene at the Royal Infirmary in the hope that it would minimize incidences of hospitalism. "Cleanliness" in hospitals often meant no more than sweeping floors and opening windows in the operating theater, and the Royal Infirmary was no exception. Lister suspected that if he could make the wards cleaner, his patients might stop dying.

And so he began subscribing to what was known in the 1860s as the "cleanliness and cold water" school of thought, which drew analogies between the tarnishing of silver and the infections caused by bad air. Advocates of this philosophy knew that if a person dipped a spoon in cold water, it would delay the formation of a sulfide coating. Using that same logic, they thought that by boiling water and letting it cool before washing both the instruments and the wound site, a surgeon could prevent postoperative infections from developing. Their emphasis on cold water specifically was meant to counteract the heat that they believed caused inflammation and fever.

Lister's focus on cleanliness was still linked to his belief that outbreaks of hospitalism were due to the poisonous atmosphere on the wards. Others had already started to question this theory. Between 1795 and 1860, three doctors put forward the idea that puerperal (or childbed) fever—which, like sepsis, was accompanied by both localized and systemic inflammation—was caused not by miasma but by *materies morbi* (morbid substances) transmitted from doctor to patient. Each believed the disease could be prevented by following strict rules of cleanliness in the hospitals.

The first of these three doctors was a Scotsman named Alexander Gordon, who was working in Aberdeen when a prolonged outbreak began there in December 1789. Over the course of three years, Gordon treated seventy-seven women who had contracted puerperal fever, twenty-five of whom died in his care. In his report published in 1795, he argued that "the cause of the epidemic Puerperal Fever under consideration was not owing to a noxious constitution of the atmosphere" [that is, miasma] but rather to the medical staff itself, which spread the fever to new patients after attending those afflicted with it. Gordon was convinced that the cause of puerperal fever was something on the practitioners themselves. He claimed he could "foretell what women would be affected with the disease, upon hearing by what midwife they were to be delivered, or by what nurse they were to be attended during their lying-in." In almost every instance, his prediction was correct. In the light of this evidence, Gordon advised that the clothing and bedsheets of the infected be burned after death and that the nurses and midwives who cared for these patients "ought carefully to wash themselves, and get their apparel properly fumigated, before it be put on again."

The second person to make this connection was the American essayist Oliver Wendell Holmes, who was also a physician and later professor of anatomy at Harvard University. In 1843, he published a pamphlet titled *The Contagiousness of Puerperal Fever*. His work was based heavily on Gordon's and laid the groundwork for a revival of the Scotsman's ideas fifty years after they were first published. Unfortunately, Holmes failed to make an impression on his contemporaries and in the 1850s was attacked for his beliefs by two prominent obstetricians, who thought it was a personal insult to be accused of being the carrier of the very disease they were trying to combat.

And then there was Ignaz Semmelweis, who solved the problem of how to prevent childbed fever in Vienna at the same time Holmes was writing about it in America. Semmelweis, who was working as an assistant physician at the city's General Hospital, noticed a discrepancy between the hospital's two obstetric wards. One was attended by medical students, while the other was under the care of midwives and their pupils. Although each ward provided identical facilities for its patients, the one that was overseen by the medical students had a significantly higher mortality rate, by a factor of three. Those within the medical community who took notice of this imbalance attributed it to the male students' rougher handling of the patients than the female midwives', which they believed compromised the vitality of the mothers, making them more susceptible to developing puerperal fever. Semmelweis wasn't convinced.

In 1847, one of his colleagues died after cutting his hand during a postmortem examination. To his surprise, the Hungarian physician realized that the disease that had killed his friend was identical to puerperal fever. What if doctors working in the deadhouse were carrying "cadaverous particles" with them onto the wards when they assisted in the delivery of babies, and it was *this* that was causing infection rates to spike? After all, Semmelweis observed, many of these young men went directly from an autopsy to attend to the pregnant women at the hospital.

Believing that puerperal fever was caused not by miasma but by "infective material" from a dead body, Semmelweis set up a basin filled with chlorinated water in the hospital. Those passing from the dissection room to the wards were required to wash their hands before attending to living patients. Mortality rates on the medical students' ward plummeted. In April 1847, the rate was 18.3 percent. After hand-washing was instituted the following month, rates in June were 2.2 percent, followed by 1.2 percent in July and 1.9 percent in August.

Semmelweis saved many lives; however, he was not able to convince many physicians of the merits of his belief that incidences of puerperal fever were related to contamination caused through contact with dead bodies. Even those willing to carry out trials of his methods often did so inadequately, producing discouraging results. After a number of negative reviews of a book he published on the subject, Semmelweis lashed out at his critics. His behavior became so erratic and embarrassing to his colleagues that he was eventually confined to a mental institute, where he spent his final days raging about childbed fever and the doctors who refused to wash their hands.

In fact, Semmelweis's methods and theories had little impact on the medical community. Lister visited a clinic in Budapest where the beleaguered physician had recently worked, and he later reflected: "Semmelweis's name was never mentioned to me having been, as it seems, entirely forgotten in his native city as in the world at large."

Try as Lister might, none of the measures he instituted affected mortality rates, not even the improved hygiene on his wards. Patients continued to die, and there seemed to be little he could do to stop it. In one week, Lister lost five of his patients to pyemia, while a majority of the others lay ill in the same ward, suffering from hospital gangrene. His house surgeon said of Lister that a divine discontent began to possess him. His mind, he said, "worked ceaselessly in an effort to see clearly the nature of the problem to be solved." Lister's exasperation spilled over into the classroom, where he turned to his students with the question that had been haunting him for some time: "It is a common observation that, when some injury is received without the skin being broken, the patient invariably recovers and that without any severe illness. On the other hand trouble of the gravest kind is always apt to follow, even in trivial injuries, when a wound of the skin is present. How is this? The man who is able to explain this problem will gain undying fame."

Then, at the end of 1864, while Lister was struggling to prevent the deaths of his patients at the Royal Infirmary, a chemistry professor and colleague, Thomas Anderson, drew his attention to something that would help him tease out the solution to the medical riddle that consumed him. It was the latest research on fermentation and putrefaction by a French microbiologist and chemist by the name of Louis Pasteur.

8.

THEY'RE ALL DEAD

**No Scientific subject can be so important to Man as that
of his own life. No knowledge can be so incessantly
appealed to by the incidents of every day, as the
knowledge of the *processes by which he lives and acts*.**

—GEORGE HENRY LEWES

U PON INQUIRING AFTER THE WELFARE of one of his patients, a
surgeon at Guy's Hospital in London was informed by his assistant that the man in question had died. The surgeon, who had
become inured to this kind of news, replied, "Oh, very well!" He
moved on to the next ward to ask about another patient. Again, the
answer came, "Dead, sir." The surgeon paused a moment. Frustrated, he cried, "Why, they're not *all* dead?" To this, his assistant
responded, "Yes, sir, they are."

Scenes like this were playing out all over Britain. Mortality rates within hospitals had reached an all-time high by the 1860s. Efforts to clean up the wards had made little impact on incidences of hospitalism. What's more, in the past several years there had been growing disagreement within the medical community over prevailing disease theories.

Cholera, in particular, had become increasingly difficult to explain within a miasmic paradigm. There had already been three major outbreaks in recent decades that had claimed the lives of nearly 100,000 people in England and Wales alone. The disease was running rampant throughout Europe, creating in its wake a medical, political, and humanitarian crisis that could not be ignored. Although non-contagionists could point to the fact that outbreaks often occurred in filthy urban areas, they could not explain why cholera had followed lines of human communication as it spread from the Indian subcontinent, nor could they resolve why some outbreaks occurred during the winter when bad smells were minimal.

Back in the late 1840s, a physician from Bristol named William Budd argued that the disease was spread by contaminated sewage carrying "a living organism of a distinct species, which was taken by the act of swallowing it, which multiplied in the intestine by self propagation." In an article published in the *British Medical Journal*, Budd wrote that "there was no proof whatever" that "the poisons of specific contagious diseases ever originate spontaneously" or were transmitted through the air via miasma. During the latter outbreak, he prioritized disinfecting measures with an antiseptic, advising, "All discharges from the sick men to be received, on their issue from the body, if possible, into vessels containing a solution of chloride of zinc."

Budd wasn't the only one to question the spontaneous origin and aerial transmission of cholera's spread. The surgeon John Snow also began investigating the matter when a deadly outbreak occurred near his house in Soho, London, in 1854. Snow started plotting cases on a map, and that was when he noticed that a majority of people who fell ill were receiving their water from a pump on the southwest corner of the intersection of Broad (now Broadwick) Street and Cambridge (now Lexington) Street. Even cases that were at first glance unconnected with the pump turned out to be associated with it after all, such as that of the fifty-nine-year-old woman who lived quite a distance from the water supply. When Snow interviewed her son, he was told that his mother often visited Broad Street because she preferred the taste of water from that particular pump. She was dead within two days of drinking from the supply.

Like Budd, Snow concluded that cholera was transmitted through contaminated water supplies, not by poisonous gases or miasmas in the air. He published a map of the epidemic to support his theory. Despite strong skepticism from the local authorities, Snow was able to persuade them to remove the handle from the Broad Street pump, after which the outbreak quickly subsided.

Incidences like this began to call into question the predominant belief within the medical community that disease arose from filth and was transmitted through the air by noxious gases, or miasmas. More proof came in 1858 when a terrible, inescapable stench crept through the city of London, pervading every nook and cranny within a mile of the river Thames. The scorching summer heat intensified the foul odor. People went out of their way to avoid coming in contact with the river. "The Great Stink" arose from human excrement piled along the riverbanks—a problem that had been growing worse as London became more and more populated. As the scientist Michael Faraday, famed for his work on electromagnetism, observed, "The feculence rolled up in clouds so dense that they were visible at the surface." As he sailed down the river one afternoon, he noted that the water was an "opaque pale brown fluid." The smell was so bad that members of Parliament had to cover their windows with heavy cloth just so they could continue working. *The Times* reported that government officials, "bent upon investigating the matter to its very depth, ventured into the library, [where they were] instantaneously driven to retreat, each man with a handkerchief to his nose."

Londoners assumed that the "poisonous effluvia" (that is, miasma) arising from the water would lead to an outbreak of disease in the city. There were even rumors that a boatman had already died from inhaling the noxious vapors. Thousands fled the city in fear for their lives. After years of trying to secure funding for a new sewer system in London, hygiene reformers thought it would be poetic if Parliament was finally made to interfere because of its own decimation. And yet, strangely, no epidemics occurred that summer.

There was a perceptible shift away from miasma and toward contagion theories in the 1850s and 1860s, due in part to these events. Many doctors, however, remained unconvinced. Snow's investigations in particular still didn't suggest a plausible mechanism for the *transmission* of the disease. His conclusions correlated cholera with contaminated drinking water. But, like other contagionists, Snow didn't explicitly state what it was that was being transmitted through that water. Was it an animalcule? Or a poisonous chemical? If the latter, wouldn't it be infinitely diluted in large bodies of water like the river Thames? What's more, Snow himself acknowledged that contagionism didn't provide a satisfactory explanation of *all* diseases, and he continued to allow for the possibility of spontaneous generation in the development of diseases that caused putrefaction, like erysipelas.

The voices crying out for a better explanation of contagious and epidemic diseases were growing ever louder.

• • •

The problem of hospital infection had vexed Lister for so long that he wondered if he would ever find a solution to it. But since his conversation with Professor Anderson about Pasteur's latest research on fermentation, he felt a renewed optimism. Lister immediately sought out Pasteur's publications on the decomposition of organic material, and with the help of Agnes he began replicating the French scientist's experiments in his laboratory at home. For the first time, the answer was within his reach.

The research with which Lister was familiarizing himself began nine years earlier when a local wine merchant approached Pasteur with a problem. Monsieur Bigo had been manufacturing wine from beetroot juice when he noticed that a large number of his vats were turning sour while they fermented. Pasteur was then dean of the Faculty of Sciences at Lille University. His reputation as a brilliant chemist had been established years earlier when he demonstrated that a crystal's shape, its molecular structure, and its effect on polarized light were all interconnected. He soon formed the view that only living agents could produce optically active asymmetric compounds and that further study of molecular asymmetry would unlock the secrets to the origin of life.

But why would Bigo consult a chemist with his problems? At the time, fermentation was thought to be a chemical process rather than a biological one. Although many scientists recognized that yeast acted as a catalyst in the conversion of sugar to alcohol, most believed that yeast was a complex chemical substance. Bigo had become acquainted with Pasteur's work because his son was one of Pasteur's students at the university. So it seemed only natural to Bigo that he should turn to the chemist for help.

In fact, Pasteur had his own reasons for wanting to investigate the causes behind the spoiled vats of wine. For some time, he had been interested in the nature of amyl alcohol, which he discovered was a "complex milieu composed of two isomers; one, which . . .

rotates the plane of light under the polarimeter; the other, which is inactive [and] has no optical activity." Moreover, the former contained the same asymmetrical characteristics that Pasteur had shown could only arise from *living* agents. Beetroot juice contained a mixture of both the inactive and the active amyl alcohols and therefore presented Pasteur with a unique opportunity to study the two isomers under different conditions.

Pasteur began making daily visits to the winery, where he eventually transformed the cellar into a makeshift laboratory. Like Bigo, he noticed that some batches of wine smelled fine, while others emanated an almost putrid odor. These vats were also covered in a mysterious film. Puzzled by this, Pasteur took samples from each of the vats and examined them under his microscope. Much to his surprise, he discovered that the shape of the yeast was different depending on the sample. If the wine was unspoiled, the yeast was round. If it was corrupted, the yeast was elongated and appeared alongside other, smaller, rod-shaped structures: bacteria. A biochemical analysis of the spoiled batches also revealed that under the wrong conditions, hydrogen attached itself to the nitrates in the beetroot, producing lactic acid, which gave off the fetid odor and made the wine taste sour.

Crucially, Pasteur was able to show that the amyl alcohol that was optically active had arisen as a result of the yeast, not from the sugar, as some scientists had previously argued. He did this by demonstrating that when measured under a polarimeter, amyl alcohol differed too much to have inherited its asymmetry from sugar, a nonliving agent. And because Pasteur believed that life alone was responsible for asymmetry, he had to conclude that fermentation was a biological process and that the yeast that helped produce wine was a living organism.

Pasteur's opponents pointed out that yeast was not required in sugar fermentations that produced lactic or butyric acid, nor was it possible to see yeast organisms in putrefying meat. But it wasn't the yeast that was responsible for the *spoiling* of the vats; rather, it was bacteria (the rod-shaped microbes) that caused the wine to go bad. In a similar vein, Pasteur also demonstrated that the same was true in sour milk and rancid butter, though the microbes responsible in each case were different from one another. There seemed to be a specificity to the properties of the microbes that he was observing under the microscope.

Pasteur's conclusions were bold. To say that the yeast acted on the beetroot juice because it was a living organism was to go against the very tenets of mainstream chemistry in the mid-nineteenth century. While the guardians of the old paradigm were willing to accept the presence of microorganisms in fermentable substances, they only did so on the basis that these microorganisms arose spontaneously as part of the fermenting process. Nevertheless, Pasteur believed that these microbes were carried through the air on dust particles and that they were born of themselves. They did not come into existence de novo.

In a series of experiments, Pasteur boiled fermentable substances to rid them of any existing microorganisms. He then placed these substances in two different kinds of flasks. The first was an ordinary flask with an open top. The second had a neck shaped like an S that prevented dust and other particles from entering the flask. This flask also remained open and exposed to the air. After a certain amount of time, the first flask began to teem with microbial life, while the swan-neck flask remained uncontaminated. From these experiments, Pasteur finally proved that microbes were not generated spontaneously; otherwise, the flask with the curved neck would have become reinfected. His experiments established what is now considered one of the cornerstones of biology: Only life begets life. In a speech on his findings delivered to the Sorbonne, Pasteur said, "Never will the doctrine of spontaneous generation recover from the mortal blow of this simple experiment." It wasn't long before the word "germ" was being used to describe these protean microbes.

In an instant, Pasteur went from being a serious chemist held in esteem by most of the scientific community to being considered a maverick by his championing of what he called "the world of the infinitely small." His research immediately fell under attack, threatening to topple long-established views of how the world worked. The scientific journal *La Presse* passed damning judgment on the French scientist: "I am afraid that the experiments you quote, M. Pasteur, will turn against you. . . . The world into which you wish to take us is really too fantastic."

Undeterred, Pasteur began to make connections between fermentation and putrefaction. "The applications of my ideas are immense," he wrote in 1863. "I am ready to approach the great mystery of the putrid diseases, which constantly occupy my mind." There was good reason for Pasteur to be so preoccupied with the subject of infectious diseases: between 1859 and 1865, three of his daughters died of typhoid fever.

Pasteur believed that putrefaction, like fermentation, was also caused by the growth of minute microorganisms that were carried through the air by dust. "Life directs the work of death at every stage," he wrote. There was just one problem, however. Pasteur was not a physician, a point he lamented as his research into the matter progressed: "How I wish I had . . . the special knowledge I need to launch myself wholeheartedly into the experimental study of one of the contagious diseases." Fortunately for Pasteur, his work had already begun to attract the attention of a select few within the medical community, like Sir Thomas Spencer Wells, surgeon to Queen Victoria.

Wells spoke of Pasteur's latest work on fermentation and putre-faction in an address to the British Medical Association in 1863, a year before it came to Lister's attention. In it, Wells argued that Pasteur's research on the decomposition of organic material shed light on the causes of putrid infections: "[By] applying the knowl-edge for which we are indebted to Pasteur of the presence in the atmosphere of organic germs . . . it is easy to understand that some germs find their most appropriate nutriment in the secretions from wounds, or in pus, and that they so modify it as to convert it into a poison when absorbed." Unfortunately, Wells failed to make the impact he had hoped at the convention. His peers were not con-vinced by the existence of germs, and like others who read Pasteur's work, Wells made no real attempt to put the germ theory of putre-faction into practice.

Lister picked up the baton. Initially, he focused on the parts of Pasteur's research that confirmed for him a view he already held: that the danger was indeed present in the air around the patient. Like Wells, Lister took away from Pasteur's work the idea that it wasn't the air as such but its constituent of microbial life that was the source of hospital infection. In those early days, he probably thought that the contamination of the air and the infection of the wound were attributable to the invasion of a single organism. Lister could not yet conceive of the vast number of airborne germs and their varying degrees of virulence, nor did he understand that germs could be transmitted in many different ways and by many different media.

Lister came to the vital realization that he couldn't prevent a wound from having contact with germs in the atmosphere. So he turned his attention to finding a means of destroying microorganisms within the wound itself, before infection could set in. Pasteur had con-ducted a number of experiments that demonstrated that germs could be destroyed in three ways: by heat, by filtration, or by antiseptics. Lister ruled out the first two because neither were applicable to the treatment of wounds. Instead, he focused on finding the most effective antiseptic for killing germs without causing further injury: "When I read Pasteur's article, I said to myself: just as we can destroy lice on the nit-filled head of a child by applying a poison that causes no lesion to the scalp, so I believe that we can apply to a patient's wounds toxic products that will destroy the bacteria without harming the soft parts of this tissue."

Surgeons had been using antiseptics to irrigate wounds for some time. The problem was that there was no consensus among doctors on what caused sepsis, and generally these substances were used to control suppuration only *after* infection had set in. Around this time, *The Lancet* reported, "It was a great part of the care of the old practitioners to avert inflammation and . . . to treat it. We are not so fearful of it now. Blood-poisoning is to surgeons of the present day as great a source of dread as inflammation was to their predecessors, and is a far larger and more real evil." Unfortunately, while blood poisoning is far more dangerous than inflammation, the medical journal got it fundamentally wrong: inflammation accompanies suppuration, which is often a *symptom* of blood poisoning and septicemia. Inflammation is not a disease in and of itself, and it often signifies that something more sinister is going on. Until this distinction was made, it was difficult for surgeons to understand the rationale behind using antiseptics before infection set in, especially because many in the medical community believed inflammation and pus were integral parts of the healing process. Good, clean, and limited laudable pus was necessary for normal wound healing, but excessive or contaminated pus was seen to be a dangerous medium for putrefaction.

Complicating matters was the fact that many antiseptic substances also proved ineffective or caused further damage to the tissue, thus making the wound even more vulnerable to infection. Everything from wine and quinine to iodine and turpentine had been used to treat infected wounds, but none proved consistently effective in stopping putrid suppuration once it had already begun. Corrosive substances like nitric acid, which could effectively combat putrefactive infection, were often diluted too much to be of any real use.

In the first few months of 1865, Lister tested many antiseptic solutions while trying to find the best one to counteract the microbes that he now understood were the cause of hospital infections. Most of these had a bad track record, possibly because they had only been employed after inflammation and suppuration had already set in. Lister wanted to test their efficacy by using these solutions prophylactically. He turned first to one of the most popular substances at this time, called Condy's fluid, or potassium permanganate, which was also used as a flash powder by early photographers. Lister tested Condy's fluid on a patient shortly after an operation, before infection had a chance to set in. His dresser, Archibald Malloch, wrote that he "held the limb in one hand, and the flaps, from which all the stitches had been cut out, in the other, while Mr. Lister poured kettle after kettleful of hot diluted Condy's fluid between the flaps to cleanse them; the stumps being finally covered with a linseed poultice." Despite the compound's having a strong oxidizing agent that could act like an antiseptic, the wound eventually began to suppurate. Lister wasn't achieving the results he sought and abandoned his trial.

Then, one day, Lister remembered reading that engineers at a sewage works in Carlisle had used carbolic acid to counteract the smell of rotting garbage and to render odorless nearby pastures that were irrigated with liquid waste. They had done this at the recommendation of Frederick Crace Calvert, an honorary professor of chemistry at the Royal Institution of Manchester, who was first introduced to the compound's miraculous properties while studying in Paris. An unexpected benefit of the engineers' efforts was that the carbolic acid also killed the protozoan parasites that had caused outbreaks of cattle plague in the livestock that grazed in these fields. Lister wrote that he was "struck with an account of the remarkable effects produced by carbolic acid upon the sewage of the town." Could this be the antiseptic he had been searching for?

Carbolic acid, also known as phenol, is a derivative of coal tar. It was first discovered in 1834 and used in its raw state as creosote to preserve railway ties and ships' timbers. It was unknown in British surgery. More often than not, it was recommended indiscriminately, sometimes as a preservative of food, sometimes as a parasiticide, sometimes as a deodorant.

Lister obtained a sample of the crude acid from the ever-resourceful Thomas Anderson and observed its properties under the microscope. He soon realized that he would need a lot more of the compound in order to test its efficacy on patients. Anderson put him in direct contact with Calvert up in Manchester, who had just started manufacturing the acid on a small scale in the form of white crystals that liquefied when heated. Calvert had long been an advocate of the use of coal tar in medicine, particularly with regard to the sloughing of wounds and the preserving of corpses for dissection. He eagerly supplied Lister with a sample of his carbolic acid.

Lister didn't have to wait long before he was able to test it on a subject. In March 1865, he carried out an excision of caries (decaying bone) from a patient's wrist at the Royal Infirmary. Afterward, he carefully washed the wound with carbolic acid, hoping it would debride it of any contaminants. Much to his dismay, infection set in, and Lister was forced to admit that the trial had been a failure. Another opportunity presented itself a few weeks later when a twenty-two-year-old named Neil Kelly was brought to the Royal Infirmary with a broken leg. Once more, Lister applied Calvert's carbolic acid to the injured limb—and suppuration soon appeared. But Lister still believed that carbolic acid was the key and blamed himself for the failure: "It proved unsuccessful, in consequence, as I now believe, of improper management."

Lister needed to implement a better system if he was going to continue trying carbolic acid on patients. He couldn't just test it haphazardly, because there were too many variables from case to case preventing him from understanding the substance's true efficacy. For that reason, he ruled out surgical cases for the time being. And because simple fractures did not involve a tear in the skin, he reasoned that microbes could not gain access by any channel other than an open wound. He decided to limit his trials of carbolic acid to compound fractures: injuries in which splintered bone lacerated the skin. This particular kind of break had a high rate of infection and frequently led to amputation. From an ethical standpoint, testing carbolic acid on compound fractures was sound. If the antiseptic failed, the leg could still be amputated—something that would have likely occurred anyway. But if the carbolic acid worked, then the patient's limb would be saved.

Lister was cautiously optimistic about this approach. All he had to do was wait for someone with a compound fracture to arrive at his hospital.

———

THE RATTLING AND RUMBLING of carriages down the busy streets of Glasgow began at sunrise and didn't stop until most of the city's occupants had gone to bed. Top-heavy stagecoaches moved precariously along uneven roads, while omnibuses packed with passengers clattered through congested thoroughfares. Hackney carriages trundled at a stately pace, and tradesmen's carts piled high with goods zigzagged through the traffic in a mad dash to supply the marketplaces. Occasionally, a hearse draped in black with its procession of mourners would slow the tumult to a respectful crawl, but most days the roads were a bustling river of wheeled and pedestrian traffic. Overcrowded cities like Glasgow sounded "as if all the noises of all the wheels of all the carriages in creation were mingled and ground together in one subdued hoarse, moaning hum," one contemporary wrote. The city's everyday cacophony was an assault on the eyes and ears of the uninitiated.

It was into this chaos that eleven-year-old James Greenlees stepped one humid day in early August 1865. He had crossed these streets countless times, but for a moment his attention had wandered. No sooner had he stepped into the traffic than a cart came crashing past him, throwing him to the ground and crushing his left leg under one of its metal-rimmed wheels. The driver halted the cart and jumped down in panic. Onlookers rushed to the scene of the accident. Greenlees lay there screaming, tears streaming down his face. His tibia had cracked under the weight of the cart and was protruding through a bleeding gash in his shin. If there was any hope of saving his leg, he would need to get to the hospital quickly.

It wasn't easy getting Greenlees to the Royal Infirmary in his condition. The heavy cart had to be moved off his leg, and he had to be gingerly lifted onto a makeshift stretcher and carried across the city. He arrived at the Royal Infirmary three hours after the accident. By the time he was admitted to the wards, Greenlees had lost a lot of blood, and the situation was critical.

As one of the surgeons on duty that afternoon, Lister was alerted to the case as soon as the boy was brought into the hospital. Lister remained calm while assessing the situation. The break was not clean. Even more worryingly, the open wound on Greenlees's leg was contaminated with dirt and dust from the journey across town. Amputation could not be ruled out. Lister knew that many patients had lost their lives because of compound fractures that were far less severe than the one this boy had endured. His father-in-law, James Syme, would probably have operated immediately. But Lister also recognized that Greenlees was very young. Losing a leg would almost certainly relegate the boy to the status of a second-class citizen, severely limiting his job opportunities in the future. How would the boy earn a living if he couldn't walk?

And yet the hard truth remained: delaying amputation would undoubtedly put Greenlees's life in danger. If the boy developed a hospital infection as a result, sawing off his leg afterward might not be enough to stop the relentless pursuit of sepsis once it took hold. At the same time, Lister still believed that carbolic acid could stave off infection, and if it did, Greenlees's leg—and his livelihood— could be saved. This was the opportunity he had been waiting for. Lister made a split-second decision. He would take his chances with the antiseptic.

Acting quickly, he administered chloroform to the boy, who at that point was delirious with pain. The open wound on Green- lees's leg had been exposed for hours. He needed to clean out the bloody gash before any microbes that had already gotten into the open- ing had a chance to multiply. With the help of his house surgeon Dr. MacFee, Lister began washing the wound thoroughly with carbolic acid. He then covered it with putty so that the solution could not be washed away by any discharges of blood and lymph. Finally, he placed a tin cap over the dressing to stop the carbolic acid from further evaporating.

Over the next three days, Lister managed Greenlees's recovery, lifting the cap and pouring more carbolic acid on the dressing to flush the wound every few hours. Greenlees was in good spirits despite the trauma he had just experienced, and Lister noted that his appetite was normal. Most important, Lister detected no rancid smell ema- nating from the dressings when he inspected the boy's leg each day. The wound was healing cleanly.

On the fourth day, Lister removed the bandages. He wrote in his casebooks that the skin had a slight blush of redness around the wound but that no suppuration was present. The fact that there was no pus was a good sign. But the redness bothered Lister. The carbolic acid was clearly irritating the boy's skin and creating the very type of inflammation that Lister was desperately trying to avoid. How could he counteract this side effect without undercutting the carbolic acid's power as an antiseptic?

Lister tried diluting the carbolic acid with water for the following five days. Unfortunately, this did little to offset the irritation caused by the antiseptic. So Lister turned to olive oil to dilute the chemical compound. This appeared to have a soothing effect on the wound without compromising the antiseptic qualities of the carbolic acid. Soon, the redness on Greenlees's leg faded, and the wound began closing up. The new solution had done the trick.

Six weeks and two days after the cart had shattered his lower leg, James Greenlees walked out of the Royal Infirmary.

Now confident that the carbolic acid was the antiseptic he had been looking for all along, Lister treated patient after patient at the Royal Infirmary using similar methods over the coming months. There was a thirty-two-year-old laborer whose right tibia was shattered after a horse kicked him, and a twenty-two-year-old factory worker whose leg was smashed to pieces after an iron box weighing 1,350 pounds slipped from its chains four feet above him. One of the more heartbreaking cases involved a ten-year-old boy who was working in a factory when he got his arm caught in a steam-powered machine. Lister reported that the boy cried out for assistance but no one came to his aid for two minutes. Meanwhile, the machine continued to move, "cutting into the ulnar side of the forearm, breaking through [the bone] about its middle, while the radius was bent [backward]." The boy was taken to the Royal Infirmary, at which point the upper fragment of his bone was protruding through the skin and two strips of muscle two to three inches in length were hanging out of the gaping wound. Lister was able to save the boy's arm, as well as his life.

It wasn't all smooth sailing. Lister experienced two failures at this time. One was a seven-year-old boy whose leg had been run over by a crowded omnibus. He developed hospital gangrene after Lister went on a vacation and handed over his care to Dr. MacFee, who was not as scrupulous as Lister in his management of the wound. The boy ultimately survived, minus one limb. The other died suddenly, weeks after he incurred his original injury. "Some days later," Lister wrote, "a very profuse haemorrhage occurred, the blood soaking through the bed, and dropping upon the floor beneath" before it came to the attention of the medical staff. It turned out that a sharp bone fragment from the man's leg fracture had pierced the popliteal artery in his thigh, causing the fifty-seven-year-old laborer to bleed to death.

Of ten compound fractures that came under his care at the hospital in 1865, eight recovered with the aid of carbolic acid. If one discounts the amputation that occurred under Dr. MacFee's care, Lister's failure rate was 9 percent. If the amputation is counted, his failure rate was 18 percent. For Lister, it was an unqualified success.

In his typical way, Lister felt it was important to be as thorough as possible and wanted to assess the efficacy of carbolic acid on other types of wounds before announcing his findings. The ultimate test would be whether Lister's methods would work on operative cases. It had been twenty years since he had witnessed Robert Liston's historic operation with ether that signaled a new age of painless surgery. Since then, surgeons had become daring with regard to how deep into the body they were prepared to cut. As operations became more invasive, postoperative infection became more and more likely. If Lister could reduce or eliminate this threat, it would change the nature of surgery forever by allowing the surgeon to perform increasingly complex operations without fear of the patient's wounds developing sepsis.

He first turned his attention to abscesses, particularly those that arose as a complication of spinal tuberculosis. Known as psoas abscesses, these develop when a large amount of pus collects on one of the long muscles in the back of the abdominal cavity. They usually grow so large that they begin to distend into the groin, requiring incision and drainage. Given the area of the body in which they form, however, psoas abscesses are prone to infection, and surgical intervention was extremely dangerous.

Over the coming months, Lister developed a technique for disinfecting the skin around the incision with carbolic acid and then dressing the cavity with a puttylike substance similar to the one he used on Greenlees. He mixed ordinary whiting (carbonate of lime) with a solution of carbolic acid in boiled linseed oil. Between the wound and the putty, he placed a piece of lint that had also been soaked in carbolic oil. The blood that soaked through the lint formed a crust underneath it. The dressing was changed daily, but the piece of oiled lint was left in place. When it came time to remove it, there was a firm cicatrix, or scar, left behind. In a letter to his father, Lister boasted: "[The] course run by cases of abscess treated in this way is so *beautifully* in harmony with the theory of the whole subject of suppuration, and besides the treatment is now rendered so simple and easy for *any* one to put in practice, that it really charms me."

In July 1866—while Lister was still refining his methods with carbolic acid—he discovered that the chair of systematic surgery at UCL was vacant. Although things were going well in Glasgow, Lister still yearned to return to his alma mater so that he could be closer to his father, who was now eighty years old. Making the prospect all the more attractive to him was the fact that the professorship also came with a permanent post at University College Hospital, where he had started his career.

Lister wrote to Lord Brougham, the president of both UCL and the hospital, asking him to support his candidacy. Accompanying his letter was the printed "Notice of a New Method of Treating Compound Fractures." In it, Lister supported the germ theory of putrefaction. Outside his own circle of friends, family, and colleagues, this was Lister's first announcement of his antiseptic principle. Shortly after he appealed to Lord Brougham for support, Lister was notified that he had lost the election. Yet Lister didn't let this news distract him from his research for long. "I have been sometimes thinking lately that I could not have been working thus had I been at University College," Lister wrote to Joseph Jackson a short while after he had received his rejection notice. "I am probably employed here much more usefully, though more quietly."

Lister returned to experimenting with carbolic acid, expanding treatment to include lacerated and contused wounds. In one instance, he removed a large tumor from a man's arm. It was situated so deeply that Lister believed the wound would have suppurated had it not been for the employment of his antiseptic system. The man escaped with both his life and his arm when he left the hospital a few weeks later.

The implications of his methods began to dawn on Lister as each year provided more proof that they worked. "I now perform an operation for the removal of a tumour, etc., with a totally different feeling from what I used to have; in fact, surgery is becoming a different thing altogether," he wrote to his father one day. If Lister could convince the world of the efficacy of his techniques, then the possibilities for the future of his profession were endless.

And so it came to be that two years after he began experimenting with carbolic acid at the Glasgow Royal Infirmary, Lister published his findings in *The Lancet*. On March 16, 1867, the first installment of a five-part article titled "On a New Method of Treating Compound Fracture, Abscess, etc., with Observations on the Conditions of Suppuration" appeared in print. The other four followed in the coming weeks and months. In these articles, Lister demonstrated that he had instituted a system based on Louis Pasteur's highly contested view that putrefaction was caused by germs in the air. He wrote that the "minute particles suspended in [the air], which are the germs of various low forms of life, long since revealed by the microscope, and regarded as merely accidental concomitants of putrescence," had now been shown by Pasteur to be its "essential cause." It was necessary to "dress the wound with some material capable of killing these septic germs." Lister's system involved using the antiseptic properties of carbolic acid in order to prevent germs from entering wounds, as well as destroying those that had already invaded the body.

His articles were instructive rather than theoretical, though his commitment to Pasteur's scientific tenets was clear. The majority of each paper laid out detailed case histories in which Lister spoke about his struggles to prevent or control putrefaction in the wounds of each patient. His intent was to *show* the readers, who were invited to feel that they were standing at Lister's shoulder, how to replicate his methods. Throughout the series of articles, he also demonstrated how his system evolved by explaining why he rejected certain types of dressings and why he tried different approaches when others had failed. The unashamedly scientific method Lister had applied to his experiments was plain for all to see.

Also evident was Lister's laudably altruistic purpose in discovering and then advocating his antiseptic method. Evincing the selflessness inculcated in him by his Quaker upbringing, he wrote: "[The] benefits which attend this practice are so remarkable that I feel it incumbent upon me to do what I can to diffuse them." Anyone seeking physical proof of these benefits could find it on his two wards at the Glasgow Royal Infirmary. Though these had previously been among the unhealthiest in the hospital due to their having limited access to fresh air, he reported that his use of antiseptic treatment on patients had greatly reduced the number suffering from infection. Not a single instance of pyemia, gangrene, or erysipelas had occurred on Lister's wards since he had introduced his system.

Lister made the first step in evangelizing for the antiseptic methods that he felt certain held the key to saving countless lives. But any sense of satisfaction would soon be tempered by troubles close to home.

9.

THE STORM

—

**Medical disputes . . . are the inevitable accidents of
scientific progress. They are like storms which purify the
atmosphere; we must be resigned to them.**

—JEAN-BAPTISTE BOUILLAUD

A S SHE STEPPED FROM THE HACKNEY CARRIAGE onto the front step of the two-story Georgian home in the summer of 1867, Isabella Pim felt the weight of the world on her shoulders. She had traveled nearly four hundred miles through the stifling summer heat to stand before this door. A few weeks earlier, Isabella—or "B.," as she was affectionately referred to by members of her family—had found a hard mass in her breast. Fearing the worst, she decided to make the arduous train journey to Glasgow by way of Edinburgh, to consult the best surgeon she knew: her brother Joseph Lister.

The sad truth was that most women of this era waited too long to seek help after finding a breast lump. During the first stages of breast cancer, the tumor is relatively painless. But surgery was an extremely painful option, and a woman would likely die even after submitting to the knife, because most surgeons didn't remove enough tissue from the breast to stop the cancer's progress. One of the most renowned surgeons in London, James Paget, lamented that cancer often returned even after he had cut away the diseased parts. "All that is locally wrong may be removed," he wrote, "but something remains, or, after a time, is renewed, and similar disease reappears and, in some form or degree, is usually worse than the first, and always tending towards death."

The risk that cancerous tissue would be left behind during an operation was especially high before anesthetics in the earlier part of the century, when such an agonizing procedure had to be performed as quickly as possible. In a letter to her daughter, sixty-year-old Lucy Thurston described the horrific ordeal that she endured during her mastectomy. When the surgeon arrived, he opened his hand to show her the knife:

> Then came a gash long and deep, first on one side of my
> breast, then on the other. Deep sickness seized me, and
> deprived me of my breakfast. This was followed by
> extreme faintness. My sufferings were no longer local.
> There was a general feeling of agony throughout the whole
> system. I felt, every inch of me, as though flesh was
> failing. . . . I myself fully intended to have seen the thing
> done. But on recollection, every glimpse I happened to
> have, was the doctor's right hand completely covered with

blood, up to the very wrist. He afterwards told me, that at one time the blood from an artery flew into his eyes, so that he could not see. It was nearly an hour and a half that I was beneath his hand, in cutting out the entire breast, in cutting out the glands beneath the arm, in tying the arteries, in absorbing the blood, in sewing up the wound, in putting on the adhesive plasters, and in applying the bandage.

Thurston survived the operation and went on to live another twenty-two years, but many did not.

With the dawn of anesthetics, breast operations became steadily more invasive now that pain was no longer a check upon the surgeon's knife. This had its own dire impact on mortality rates, for various reasons. In 1854, Alfred Armand Velpeau—the lead surgeon at the University of Paris—urged his surgical colleagues to treat breast cancer more aggressively to ensure that all the cancerous tissue was excised. To do this, he suggested that not only the breast but also the underlying chest muscles be removed in what is known as an en bloc mastectomy. This, of course, left the patient vulnerable to infection afterward.

Isabella now found herself facing a similar dilemma. A surgeon at St. Bartholomew's Hospital in London had already refused to operate, and during her stopover in Edinburgh, James Syme also advised against a mastectomy. The tumor was large, and it would require extensive removal of tissue if the surgery was to be effective. Even if Isabella survived the operation, Syme was concerned that the open chest wound would become septic and that she would die. Although he had employed Lister's antiseptic system successfully on his own patients, Syme still worried that a wound of this size would be difficult to manage with or without carbolic acid.

Better to live out the remaining time she had, of whatever duration that might be.

But Isabella had not yet abandoned hope. She knew that her brother had removed many cancerous tumors in his lifetime. More recently, she had heard from her brother that he had reduced the risk of postoperative infection through the use of carbolic acid. As Lister wrote, "B. seems to have thorough confidence in me."

After examining Isabella, Lister agreed to perform what would be his first mastectomy. In so doing, he was going against the medical advice of two well-respected men in his profession. But if there was a small chance he could stop the cancer from spreading deeper into his beloved sister's body, he had to try. "Considering *what* the operation is to be," he wrote to his father, "I would rather not let anyone else do it." Not that anyone else had volunteered.

First he visited the dissection room at the university, where he practiced the mastectomy on a corpse. Just as he was steeling himself to operate, however, he decided at the eleventh hour to visit Edinburgh to consult with Syme. Clearly, the fact that a man whose counsel he held in such high esteem had initially advised against the surgery was on his mind. Syme capitulated. "No one can say that the operation does not afford a chance," he told his son-in-law after a lengthy conversation. The two men discussed Lister's recent work with carbolic acid. Syme suggested that using it on Isabella might obviate much of the danger involved. "I felt his true kindness & *manifest*, though little expressed, sympathy, very much, & left Edinburgh much relieved," Lister wrote of his meeting with Syme.

With his mind somewhat at ease, he returned to Glasgow and made preparations to operate on Isabella. A day before the appointed moment, he sent a letter back home to Joseph Jackson: "I suppose before this reaches thee the operation on darling B. will be over. It was evidently undesirable to delay a day longer than was necessary as soon as it was determined that it was to be: so last evening I finally made arrangements . . . and we intend that the operation shall be at half past one o'clock to-morrow." Isabella's mastectomy would not take place at the Royal Infirmary, because this would only increase her risk of developing some form of hospital infection. Instead, Lister decided to carry out the mastectomy in his own home, using his own dining table—a common choice for those who could afford private care.

On June 16, 1867, Isabella Lister Pim entered the makeshift operating theater, where her brother was standing with three assistants. The instruments, which had been dipped in carbolic acid beforehand, were hidden underneath a cloth so she wouldn't be perturbed by the sight of them. She settled herself on the table at which she had dined just the previous evening, and before long she was in a deep slumber due to the effects of chloroform. Lister and the three surgeons proceeded to dip their hands in a solution of carbolic acid. They then cleansed the site of Isabella's operation. Lister stepped forward, knife in hand. Carefully, he divided both of the pectoral muscles and cleared out the armpit. After he had removed the breast tissue, muscles, and lymph nodes, Lister turned his attention to dressing the wound.

Lister covered her chest with eight layers of gauze that had been presoaked in an antiseptic solution consisting of carbolic acid and linseed oil. Over the course of his experiments, he had discovered that porous materials were not ideal for antiseptic dressings because the carbolic acid could be washed away by blood and discharge. He slipped a less permeable piece of cotton cloth called a jaconet—which had also been soaked in an antiseptic lotion—underneath the top layer of gauze. This enabled discharge to seep from the wound but prevented the carbolic acid from escaping with it. He applied these dressings to both her front and her back. Each strip of gauze reached from the acromion (the bony prominence at the top of the shoulder blade) to a little below the elbow and traversed the spine to the arm.

Lister also placed a substantial mass of gauze between her side and the lower part of her arm to prevent it from being too close to her body. Although the position was uncomfortable for Isabella, he believed it was especially important that the wound be nowhere near her arm so that it could drain freely. Bandaged like a mummy, Isabella was moved to a guest bedroom and left to convalesce.

His assistant Hector Cameron remarked on how much it cost Lister mentally and emotionally to undertake such a bold procedure on one so dear to him. When it was over, a sense of relief washed over Lister: "I am very glad it has been done. . . . I may say the operation was done at *least* as well as if she had not been my sister. But I do not wish to do such a thing again."

Isabella's wound healed without suppuration due to Lister's careful application of carbolic acid during and after her procedure. Because of his efforts, Isabella lived another three years before the cancer returned, this time in her liver. Unlike before, there was nothing Lister could do for her. His antiseptic system, however, brought about a new hope for the future of breast surgery. One day soon, the surgeon would be able to base his decisions to perform mastectomies on prognosis alone—not on whether a patient was at risk of developing postoperative sepsis.

Bolstered by the achievement with Isabella's mastectomy, as well as his continued success at the Royal Infirmary, Lister presented a paper about his work with carbolic acid to the British Medical Association. On August 9, 1867, he delivered the paper, titled "On the Antiseptic Principle in the Practice of Surgery." Only weeks earlier, the last article in his five-part series had appeared in *The Lancet*. As yet, there had been no negative reactions to his research by the medical community. Indeed, the response so far had been overwhelmingly positive. Syme had thrown his support behind Lister when he reported in *The Lancet* seven successful cases involving the application of carbolic acid to both compound fractures and surgery. And shortly after Lister's lecture at the British Medical Association, the editor of *The Lancet* expressed cautious optimism: "If Professor Lister's conclusions with regard to the power of carbolic acid in compound fractures should be confirmed . . . it will be difficult to overrate the importance of what we really call his discovery."

A storm was brewing, however. As the first voices of dissent arose, the initial resistance to Lister's antiseptic methods had little to do with whether they actually worked. What seemed to be the most contentious issue was that many of his critics mistakenly believed Lister was claiming credit for discovering the antiseptic qualities of carbolic acid, which surgeons on the Continent had been using for years. On September 21, a letter appeared in the Edinburgh *Daily Review*, signed by "Chirurgicus." In it, the author wrote that he feared Lister's recent article on the use of carbolic acid in surgery was "calculated to bring down on us some discredit—particularly among our French and German neighbours—in as far as it attributes the first surgical employment of carbolic acid to Professor Lister." Chirurgicus went on to point out that the French physician and pharmacist Jules Lemaire had written on carbolic acid long before Lister's first use of it: "I have . . . lying before me, a thick volume on the subject . . . written by Dr. Lemaire, of Paris, and the second edition of which was published in 1865." Lemaire had shown carbolic acid's "utility in arresting suppuration in surgery, and, as a dressing to compound fractures and wounds," the author maintained.

Although it had been written under a pseudonym, everyone knew Chirurgicus's letter had been penned by the influential doctor who had discovered chloroform, James Y. Simpson. The renowned obstetrician had enthusiastically distributed the text to people in the medical community, including to the editor of *The Lancet*, James G. Wakley. A week later, the letter appeared in the journal with an accompanying note from Wakley: "To Professor Lister is due the credit of having made the agent extensively known in this country." With these words, the world's leading medical journal had made it seem as if Lister's only achievement had been to replicate a Continental practice in Britain, when in fact he was proposing a revolutionary approach to wound management based on a scientific theory.

Simpson had his own motivations for wishing to minimize the significance of Lister's antiseptic treatment. The truth was that if Lister's methods worked, they would come into direct conflict with Simpson's technique of acupressure, which also aimed at promoting healing without suppuration. (This was the same method that Syme denounced when he shredded Simpson's pamphlet in front of an audience in the operating theater of the Royal Infirmary in Edinburgh.) Acupressure halted bleeding during surgery by using metal needles to fasten the severed ends of large blood vessels to the underside of the skin or muscular tissue, thus eliminating the need for ligatures, which often became a source of contamination after an operation. Lister had already rejected acupressure in a paper published in 1859, and Simpson could not let the slight go. The obstetrician even sent Lister a copy of his pamphlet on the technique with a covering letter criticizing the profession's "strange and inexplicable" use of ligatures that "sedulously and systematically implant[ed] . . . dead and decomposing arterial tissue in every large wound." He obsessed over the fact that so few surgeons had adopted his technique. An early biographer said that Simpson was jealous of everything that challenged acupressure: "Nothing, he thought, should be tolerated whose tendency was to continue the use of the ligature in amputations, after the superiority of acupressure had, as he believed, been established."

Lister found himself once more locking horns with the bull-headed Simpson. Several weeks after the original attack appeared in the Edinburgh *Daily Review,* Lister responded to Chirurgicus in *The Lancet.* He admitted that he had never read Lemaire's book but claimed that this was "hardly surprising," because the French surgeon's work "does not appear to have attracted the attention of our profession." He went on to defend his own system, saying that visitors to Glasgow who had seen his antiseptic treatment firsthand had not questioned its originality. "The novelty," he wrote, was "not the surgical use of carbolic acid (which I never claimed), but the methods of its employment with view of protecting the reparatory processes from disturbances by external agency." Lister ended his response with a gibe at the author: "Trusting that such unworthy cavils will not impede the adoption of a useful procedure, I am, Sir, Yours etc."

Lister sought out the book by Lemaire in order to prepare for what was to come. The seven-hundred-page volume was nowhere to be found in Glasgow, so he traveled to Edinburgh, where he obtained a copy from the university's library. It had conveniently turned up only a few days earlier—possibly placed there by Simpson himself, though Lister never voiced that suspicion. During the course of his reading, Lister discovered that Lemaire had recommended carbolic acid for nearly every conceivable ailment. Most important, he offered no method or guiding principle for its use. And while it was true that Lemaire reported the effectiveness of carbolic acid in disinfecting the atmosphere and improving the healing of wounds, he also recommended it as a means of decreasing the smell emanating from bodily discharge. He did not believe that pus was the result of corruption. After reading the book, Lister vented to his father that he was skeptical of Lemaire's claims: "I find reason to believe that he looks with most rose-coloured spectacles at the results of his experiments" because the French surgeon had used an "*extremely* weak watery solution of the acid."

On October 19, Lister published a second response to Chirurgicus.

He reiterated that he had never claimed to have been the first to use carbolic acid in surgery: "The success which has attended its employment here depends not so much on any specific virtue in it, as on the wonderful powers of recovery possessed by injured parts when efficiently protected against the pernicious influence of decomposition." Did this mean that carbolic acid wasn't the key factor driving his encouraging results? Perhaps as an attempt to steer the conversation away from Lemaire and back toward his core treatment methods, Lister claimed that had he "made the experiment with other antiseptics in ordinary use . . . I really think it likely I should have got very much the same results, had I gone upon the same principles."

Accompanying his reply was a letter that had been sent to Lister by a medical student named Philip Hair who lived in Carlisle, the same town that had treated its sewage with carbolic acid years earlier. Lister asserted that the young man had "no difficulty in distinguishing between the mere use of carbolic acid and the practice which I have recommended." In his letter, Hair testified that he had studied in Paris the previous winter and that he had seen nothing comparable to Lister's antiseptic treatment practiced there. Since his return, Hair had also witnessed Lister's techniques being used successfully in Edinburgh and wrote that he would be happy to furnish Lister with the names and addresses of eight fellow graduates who could bear testimony to his statements.

Simpson didn't like to be challenged, and Lister's reply only angered him further. The obstetrician abandoned his alias and replied to Lister directly in *The Lancet*. He began with a sarcastic reference to Lister's phrase "unworthy cavils," which all but outed him as the author of the letter in the Edinburgh *Daily Review*. Again, Simpson alluded to Lemaire and accused Lister of having almost culpable ignorance of the existing medical literature. He went on to say that William Pirrie at the University of Aberdeen Hospital had employed acupressure to stop suppuration in two-thirds of his cases involving the removal of tumors from breasts and that acupressure was the superior method for preventing the formation of pus, regardless of whether or not Lister's antiseptic treatment worked. In case no one had understood him clearly the first time, Simpson added, "Let me here take the liberty of briefly pointing out that Mr. Lister has been most undoubtedly preceded by other authors in all his leading theories and uses in connexion with this subject."

Lister didn't take the bait. He sent a short reply to *The Lancet*: "As I have already endeavoured to place the matter in its true light without doing injustice to anyone, I must forbear from any comment on [Simpson's] allegations." Instead, he told readers that he would prove the merits of his system in a series of papers that would appear in the coming months, and let the medical community decide for itself whether Simpson's criticisms were justified. Lister believed his system should be judged on its scientific evidence, not on how eloquently he defended himself.

As luck would have it, Professor Pirrie—whose name Simpson had invoked in defense of acupressure—published an article in *The Lancet* on the very day that Lister's final response appeared in the journal. Specifically, he praised the virtues of carbolic acid for treating burns and predicted that if Lister's antiseptic method was equally useful in treating other ailments, "it would be a great blessing in the treatment of these dangerous and painful injuries." Nowhere in the article did he mention acupressure. For the moment, Simpson fell quiet.

Although publicly Lister maintained a dignified silence, privately he felt wounded by the attacks. In a letter to Joseph Jackson, he wrote, "I have always felt that for the editors of these medical journals to take no notice at all of any articles I might write was the best that could happen; so that the good, if there was any, in my work might quietly produce its effect in improving the knowledge and treatment of disease." He added, mournfully, "Fame is no plant that grows on mortal soil." Lister's nephew said of his uncle that he found Simpson's attacks repugnant and distressing. The quiet, reserved surgeon—who once thought the Scottish cities would suit his temperament better than London because there were far fewer professional quarrels—was beginning to realize how difficult the task ahead would be. He would need more than the testimony of a few medical students to encourage surgeons to take his antiseptic treatment seriously.

Many opponents likened Lister's antiseptic system to the traditional practice of putting ointments on putrefactive wounds and hoping for the best—like those practitioners who had been using wine, quinine, and Condy's fluid for decades. A young physician from Liverpool named Frederick W. Ricketts sided with Simpson, arguing that acupressure was "simple, effectual, and elegant," while Lister's methods were "obsolete and inelegant." In a similar way, James Morton, a physician who had worked with Lister at the Royal Infirmary until his tenure ended in October 1867, concluded that carbolic acid was "certainly not superior, barely equal, to some of the other antiseptics in common use." Like Ricketts, Morton thought that Lister's methods were outdated and took issue with their being called a "system" of treatment. Instead, he characterized them as "an antiseptic mode of dressing"—one of many already in existence—and thought Lister had "allowed his pen to run probably a little too fast" when praising his own results.

While the older generation of surgeons were willing to try his antiseptic treatment on patients, they struggled to accept the germ theory of putrefaction, which was at the heart of his system. If surgeons continued to misunderstand the cause of infection, they were unlikely to apply his treatment correctly. In the midst of this debate, Lister presented an address to the Medico-Chirurgical Society of

Glasgow in which he emphasized that efforts in employing the anti-septic treatment should be directed on sound principles, namely, Louis Pasteur's.

Lister's colleague Morton didn't just find fault with his methods. He also didn't accept the premise that germs were to blame for putrefaction. Morton characterized Lister's published research as fearmongering. "Nature is here regarded as some murderous hag," he wrote, "whose fiendish machinations must be counteracted. She must be entrapped into good behavior, she is no longer to be trusted." Even the editor of *The Lancet* refused to use the word "germs," instead calling them "septic elements contained in the air." It was difficult for many surgeons at the height of their careers to face the fact that for the past fifteen or twenty years they might have been inadvertently killing patients by allowing wounds to become infected with tiny, invisible creatures.

There were practical problems with Lister's antiseptic treatment as well. His methods were considered overly complicated, and they were constantly evolving. Even if surgeons accepted that germs were the culprit, many of them were unable or unwilling to follow his methodology with the level of precision needed to achieve the promised results. They had been trained by a generation of surgeons who valued speed and practicality over exactitude. "Mr. Rouse has occasionally sponged the wound, in the operating theatre, before applying the sutures, but not having found any advantage arise from it, he has discontinued the practice," one report read. Similarly, Mr. Holmes Coote "does not approve of Lister's method, which he considers meddlesome." Another surgeon reported that Lister's antiseptic treatment was sufficient to destroy putrefaction once it had set in, but it was not good as a preventive measure: "Yet in regard to its antipurulent properties such satisfactory results have not been obtained."

The illustrious surgeon James Paget had also experienced mixed results using Lister's antiseptic treatment in London. In his first published article about it, he conceded that he might have been applying the system incorrectly. Within a short period, however, Paget rejected Lister's system altogether, stating that it was dangerous, especially in cases where carbolic acid was left on the wound too long. This time around, Paget claimed, he had followed each step carefully, "if not with all the skill that Professor Lister would employ it, yet with more than is ever likely to be generally used in the treatment of fractures." Lister's antiseptic treatment "certainly did no good," in Paget's opinion.

Given his prominence in the medical community, Paget's testimony was damning. It wasn't a surprise that the greatest resistance to Lister's antiseptic treatment had come from the capital. As verdict after verdict against Lister rolled in, the editor of *The Lancet* wondered why London seemed to be especially resistant to his methods. "Are the conditions of suppuration different here from those in Glasgow?" he asked facetiously. "Or is it that the antiseptic treatment is not tried with that care without which Mr. Lister has always pointed out it does not succeed?" As long as others were applying his methods shoddily or halfheartedly, winning hearts and minds would prove next to impossible. Lister needed to go with a more proactive approach.

10.

THE GLASS GARDEN

—

New opinions are always suspected, and usually opposed, without any other reason but because they are not already common.

—JOHN LOCKE

JAMES SYME CAUGHT HIS ASSISTANT giving him a peculiar look from across the room. Thomas Annandale had been watching him closely all morning while he examined patients in his consultation room at Shandwick Place, and it was beginning to grate on his nerves. The last two months had been tough on the old surgeon, and he was feeling out of sorts. It was the spring of 1869, and Syme was nearly seventy years old. His wife, Jemima, had died unexpectedly in February, leaving an empty space in his heart and his home.

Joseph Jackson—himself a widower—wrote to his son upon hearing the news: "I have truly felt for thy estimable father-in-law under his bereavement and the desolation he must feel at home." Millbank House just wasn't the same without Jemima's comforting presence.

Syme knew that his friends and his family were worried about him. But on this particular morning, he felt that Annandale's concern was more specific. An hour earlier, Syme felt his mouth twist slightly as he was speaking to a patient, and his hand shook as he scribbled out a prescription. Still, he didn't think much of it. Perhaps his stutter had momentarily returned, or maybe it was age related. Whatever the cause, though, Annandale was beginning to make him feel uneasy, and he decided to put a stop to it. In case the young man thought he hadn't noticed the little episode, Syme announced in a loud, distinct voice, "What a curious nervous feeling I had just now; I felt as if I wanted to speak and could not."

As the day wore on, Syme performed several operations around the city. All the while, he could feel Annandale's eyes boring into him. The younger surgeon positioned himself at Syme's side during each procedure. "Although I was anxiously watching every step," Annandale later said, "I could detect nothing in Mr. Syme's actions [during the operations] . . . out of the common." And yet his assistant couldn't shake the feeling that something wasn't quite right.

The two men returned to the private clinic at Shandwick Place late that afternoon. Syme's son and niece were waiting for him in his consultation room when he arrived, and he was given temporary reprieve from Annandale's critical gaze while he spoke privately with his family. After a brief but pleasant conversation, Syme ushered them out in anticipation of the arrival of his next patient. As he shut the door to his office, he noticed his assistant approach his family to speak with them quietly in the hallway.

A few minutes later, a loud crash rang out as Syme collapsed onto the floor.

• • •

Syme had suffered a paralytic stroke, and although he retained the ability to speak, he had lost the use of the left side of his body. The situation appeared grim, but those around him were optimistic. The elderly surgeon had recovered from a stroke a year earlier. Everyone assumed the outcome would be the same the second time around. *The Lancet* broke the news to the medical world, stating that the attack was not severe and "strong hopes are entertained of a complete recovery." A few weeks later, *The Lancet* again reported on Syme's health. He had regained movement in his hand and was now able to walk around his garden. "We only echo the feeling of the whole profession," the article continued, "when we express the wish that Mr. Syme may long be spared, if not to operate with his rare skill, at any rate to contribute his clearly defined opinions on those professional questions in regard to which his large experience and shrewd judgment make him an authority."

Lister and his wife traveled to Edinburgh to be with Syme while he convalesced. Agnes shared nursing duties with her younger sister Lucy, and slowly but surely, Syme began to recover. But the elder surgeon soon recognized his own limitations. That summer, he resigned his position as chair of clinical surgery at the University of Edinburgh with the hope that Lister would take his place. Shortly after, 127 medical students at the university wrote to Lister, imploring him to accept the position. "We take this step from a conviction that you are the man most capable," they wrote, "from your high attainments and achievements in Surgery, to maintain the dignity and renown which have been conferred upon the Chair and the University by Mr. Syme." They praised Lister for his contributions to science and for his recent research with carbolic acid: "Your method of Antiseptic Treatment constitutes a well-marked epoch in the history of British Surgery, and will result in lasting glory to the Profession, and unspeakable benefit to mankind." Lister needed no further persuasion. On August 18, 1869, he was elected to the chair of clinical surgery at the University of Edinburgh.

It was a felicitous return, albeit one that happened under tragic circumstances. One of Syme's friends wrote to Lister that it was a "great happiness to all—especially Mr. Syme, who I think would not have cared to live had the worst been taken and the best lost." *The Lancet* lauded the appointment, though the editors of the journal were careful not to endorse Lister's antiseptic treatment: "We have throughout strongly supported the candidature of Mr. Lister. . . . Even if the hopes which have been raised in connection with his antiseptic labours have to be qualified, he is well calculated to raise the scientific character of surgery."

The following month, Lister and Agnes moved back to Edinburgh. They took up temporary lodgings at 17 Abercromby Place before moving to a lavish house at 9 Charlotte Square. The house had once belonged to Syme before he moved to Millbank, and although committing to the property involved an enormous sum of money, Lister could afford it. He had come a long way since his days as a house surgeon.

Meanwhile, the ridicule of Lister's antiseptic system continued to grow. Many within the medical community tried to paint him as a pretentious charlatan whose ideas were foolish at best, dangerous at worst. At University College Hospital in London, the surgeon John Marshall railed against the antiseptic treatment after observing green urine in a woman who had undergone a mastectomy. Similar reports followed. These surprised Lister. He was already aware of the perils of carbolic acid poisoning, having witnessed the results of it firsthand, and years earlier had warned doctors to dilute the solution. He was certain that this was just another example of his methods failing because others were careless in how they employed them.

One of the more critical voices was that of Donald Campbell Black, a surgeon from Glasgow, who called Lister's antiseptic treatment "the latest toy of medical science." He thought Lister's results were due to coincidences and warned against what he called the "carbolic acid mania." He wrote that there was "nothing more opposed to the true progress of scientific medicine or surgery" than the "mounting hobbies" of surgeons like Lister. What's more, Black questioned whether there had actually been an improvement at the Royal Infirmary. He had acquired statistics from *The Medical Times and Gazette* that suggested there had been no change in mortality rates from amputations and compound fractures in Lister's hospital in an eight-year period.

From 1860 to 1862, one-third of those who underwent amputation died. One-fourth of those who suffered compound fractures but did not undergo amputation also died. There were similar mortality rates for 1867 and 1868, when Lister's antiseptic system had been introduced into the hospital. Indeed, there was a slight increase in the number of patients who died from amputations, though these statistics were misleading because they represented the total deaths throughout the entire hospital. Not every surgeon at the Glasgow Royal Infirmary had adopted Lister's techniques. Even among those who accepted his methods, many did not execute them with the precision and consistency needed to produce the promised results. Lister would need to distinguish his own successes from those of other surgeons within the same hospital in the future in order to address this type of discrepancy.

Those who *did* accept Lister's results still harbored doubts over the actual reasons behind the decline in mortality rates. Several doctors claimed that his success was due to overall improvements in hygiene in the new surgical building at the hospital—not just to his antiseptic system. Lister fought back: "To suppose that the kind of change which I have described as having taken place in the salubrity of my wards can be attributed to the causes referred to, is simply out of the question." He reiterated that his wards had been among the most unhealthy at Glasgow's Royal Infirmary before he began employing carbolic acid, going as far as to say it was a "questionable privilege to be connected with the institution." The blame, he believed, lay squarely with the hospital managers, the same ones who had blocked his appointment to the Royal Infirmary when he first moved to Glasgow. Lister wrote, "I engaged in a perpetual contest with the managing body, who, anxious to provide hospital accommodation for the increasing population of Glasgow . . . were disposed to introduce additional beds." Although the managers had removed a high wall on the wards to improve air circulation, this had occurred *after* he had been treating patients with carbolic acid for nine months. Therefore, Lister believed this could not have accounted for the decline in mortality rates on his wards. As to those people who attributed his success to improved diets and increased rations on his wards, Lister wrote that the idea that diet alone could abolish pyemia, erysipelas, and hospital gangrene "would hardly enter the mind of an intelligent medical man."

Lister's remarks about the state of Glasgow's Royal Infirmary did not go unnoticed by its hospital managers, many of whom already harbored disdain for the trailblazing surgeon. Henry Lamond, secretary to the directors, was quick to respond. Writing to the editor of *The Lancet*, Lamond said that Lister's accusations "so far as they relate to the alleged unhealthiness and condition of the hospital . . . are unfair and not supported by facts." The administrators believed that Lister's antiseptic treatment had contributed very little to declining mortality rates at the hospital in recent years. Instead, they maintained that "the improved health and satisfactory condition of the hospital, which has been as marked in the medical as in the surgical department, is mainly attributable to the better ventilation, the improved dietary, and the excellent nursing to which the Directors have given so much attention of late years."

The most publicly damning critique came from Thomas Nunneley, an English surgeon in Leeds who took great pride in having not permitted a single patient of his to be treated with carbolic acid. In his address to the British Medical Association in 1869, he said that Lister's antiseptic system was based on "unsupported fancies, which have little other existence than what is found in the imagination of those who believe in them." He thought that Lister's advocacy of the germ theory was preposterous: "This speculation of organic germs is, I fear, far more than an innocent fallacy," he told conference attendees, among them James Y. Simpson. "It is a positive injury," he continued, "for teaching . . . that those desperate consequences which so often follow wounds result from one cause alone, and are to be prevented by attending to it alone . . . leads to the ignoring of those many and often complicated causes."

In his response to Nunneley, Lister could barely disguise his disgust: "That he should dogmatically oppose a treatment which he so little understands; and which, by his own admission, he has never tried, is a matter of small moment." Sensing his son's growing frustration over the attacks, Joseph Jackson sought to comfort him. In a letter, he wrote, "However slowly & imperfectly the improvements suggested by thee may be adopted & however thy claims may be slighted or disputed, it is a great thing to have been permitted to be the means of introducing so great a blessing as the antiseptic Treatment to thy fellow mortals."

While Lister was fighting a war of words with skeptics, troubling news arrived from his family again. A few weeks after he moved to Edinburgh, he received a message from his brother Arthur, who had recently paid a visit to Upton to see their father. Arthur confessed that he had not been "prepared to see so great a change in dear Papa." Joseph Jackson was so weak that he barely had the strength to turn over in bed. Their father was now eighty-three years old, and while he had always been a robust man, Lister had started to notice small changes in Joseph Jackson over the last several years. He had suffered from a severe cough a few months earlier, and in one of his last letters to Lister he complained about a skin infection on his ankle. Even more telling was the fact that his father's once clear copperplate handwriting had become increasingly illegible—a sure sign that the octogenarian's coordination was beginning to fail him, just as Syme's had after the stroke.

Lister packed his bags and headed to London. He arrived in the nick of time. Five days later, on October 24, 1869, Joseph Jackson died. The loss hit Lister hard. Whenever Lister was vexed by, and uncertain of, his life and career choices, Joseph Jackson had been a guiding light and voice of reason. When Lister considered abandoning a career in medicine to become a Quaker minister, his father had foreseen that this was the wrong path for his son and gently steered him back toward the right one. Lister would miss his father's cherished counsel.

Deep in the throes of grief, Lister wrote to his brother-in-law Rickman Godlee. He described a strange dream he had on his last night in his childhood home. In the dream, Lister came down from his bedroom at Upton House and was greeted heartily by his father. "He shook me warmly by the hand and kissed me as he used to do when I was a little boy," Lister wrote. They exchanged a few words before Lister asked his father if he had slept well after his long journey. Joseph Jackson replied that he hadn't but that he was quite well, and the two rejoiced. It was then that Lister noticed that his father was clutching a little book, which he understood contained notes of

Joseph Jackson's journey. At that moment, Lister awoke and thought how interesting it would have been to read them.

He ended his letter with an earnest, almost poetic wish: "May I but meet thee on that peaceful shore."

Two weeks after his father's death, Lister delivered the introductory lecture to his new students at the University of Edinburgh. He paid homage to Syme, who was in attendance. "We may all rejoice that our master is still among us," Lister said, perhaps thinking of his own father. He told the young men who had gathered that because he had "free access to [Syme's] inexhaustible store of wisdom and experience, he will, in some sense, through me be still your teacher."

Syme's condition had been deteriorating. A few months after Lister's inaugural lecture, the old surgeon lost the ability to speak. The ability to swallow then deserted him too, which was a fatal situation in an era when feeding tubes did not exist. It was clear that Syme was not going to recover this time. On June 26, 1870, "the Napoleon of Surgery" died.

The medical world mourned the loss of such an eminent surgeon. Writers at *The Lancet* lamented, "In Mr. Syme there dies one of the compactest thinkers, and perhaps the best teacher of surgery, in the world. . . . [He] will not be forgotten while any of his pupils live, and as a surgeon he will be remembered as long as men need the art of surgery." Similarly, editors at the *British Medical Journal* said of him, "There can be no hesitation in placing Mr. Syme in the first rank amongst our modern surgeons."

Lister grieved the death more than most. He had lost two father figures within a year. And now that Syme was gone, there were few senior surgeons left with whom he could consult. Lister's nephew later said that as long as Syme lived, he would be recognized as "the first surgeon in Scotland." With his death, the nation would now look to confer that honor upon Joseph Lister.

—

SO FAR THE MEDICAL COMMUNITY seemed reluctant to accept the idea that microscopic organisms caused disease. As one of Lister's assistants astutely observed: "A new and great scientific discovery is always apt to leave in its trail many casualties among the reputations of those who have been champions of an older method. It is hard for them to forgive the man whose work has rendered their own of no account." If it was difficult for an older surgeon to "unlearn" decades of orthodoxy, Lister reasoned it would be a lot easier to convert the incoming students to his theories and methods. He had already created a dedicated following in Glasgow, and now he hoped to do the same in Edinburgh.

The principal feature of Lister's course was demonstration. His lectures often focused on theories of infection that were complemented with case histories and laboratory demonstrations. Lister offered a treasury of recommendations, warnings, and illustrations—all based on his own experiences. He even brought patients from the wards into the operating theater when he addressed his students at the hospital. Lister's goal was not to enumerate facts but to inculcate principles. One student remembered that although the subject was new to him, the "facts were so clear and logically set out that I thought there could hardly be any other side to the question." William Watson Cheyne—who would later become a celebrated surgeon and an advocate of antisepsis—remarked on the difference between Lister's course on systematic surgery and one given by another professor, when he was a student in Edinburgh. The latter consisted of "very dreary performances full of curious theories about the reactions of the body and inflammation" and were "quite unintelligible to me," he wrote. In contrast, Cheyne reported feeling "entranced by the wonderful vision laid before us by Lister" and left the lecture room on the first day of class "an enthusiast for the profession."

Lister's students expected a lot from their instructor, and he, in turn, expected much from them. He managed his classroom like a policeman. As was customary during this time, students presented tickets inscribed with their names when they attended a lecture. This allowed an instructor to note absentees. Using this system, Lister banned those who habitually missed his class. He collected admission tickets personally at the door as the young men filed into his inner sanctum. This was to ensure that students didn't submit two cards on behalf of an absent friend—a common practice that Lister abhorred. "Anything that leads a man to think it a matter of indifference whether he writes or tells a lie is most pernicious," Lister wrote; "he comes to write lies afterwards with the same indifference." He also monitored access to the classroom so that students couldn't interrupt him with tardy arrivals. "I have all the entrances or exits so arranged that nobody can come into the class-room after a certain time," he wrote, "and the students can only go out by a single door."

Many professors at the University of Edinburgh were known to lose their tempers and storm out of a classroom when they couldn't control their unruly pupils. But Lister commanded an audience in a way his colleagues did not. His classroom was a revered place where people could come to worship science. As one of his former students said, "[A] pin-drop could be heard in his presence; he riveted attention and cast a spell of seriousness and earnestness over all." Only once was that spell broken, when a young man joked in "sonorous and clerical tones" about Lister's antiseptic treatment. Lister raised his eyes to the joker and shot him a sad and pitying glance. The effect was magical, said the same student, who noted that a year later the heckler in question died of a general paralysis. "We knew nothing then of spirochetes [the bacteria responsible for syphilis] and it was playfully suggested Jove had smitten him for the sacrilege."

Lister held his surgical assistants to the same high standards that he did his students. He caused quite the scene one day when he asked his surgical dresser for a knife while attending to a patient on the wards. The dresser handed a scalpel to Lister, who carefully tested the edge of the knife against his palm and found it to be defective. Solemnly and slowly, Lister walked across the room and placed the instrument onto the fire. He repeated his request. Again the dresser handed him a scalpel, and again Lister discarded it in the fire. "The patients were amazed at the extraordinary sight of the Professor burning his instruments; the students were galvanised to attention, glancing now at Lister, then at me, and those on the outskirts of the crowd suddenly aroused to extraordinary curiosity to discover what it was all about," the dresser later wrote. Lister returned once more and asked for a knife. Fearful and trembling, the young man handed him a third scalpel. This one was finally accepted. Lister looked directly into the dresser's face before reprimanding him: "How dare you hand me a knife to use upon this poor man that you would not like to have used on yourself?"

Lister had reason to be strict with his students and his assistants. Every successful procedure and every successful application of antiseptic dressing served as evidence against the doctrine of spontaneous generation. Life did not develop de novo, as his students could plainly see when infection failed to develop. His reports in *The Lancet* might not have been enough to convince some surgeons of the validity of the germ theory, but his students saw with their own eyes the antiseptic system working every time they accompanied him onto the wards. If seeing was believing, Lister was creating a group of disciples: men who would graduate and spread his ideas beyond the narrow confines of the university. His followers, who later became known as the "Listerians," soon came to dominate the institutions and ideology of British surgery, spreading the doctrine of antisepsis with a reverential devotion.

The announcement of Lister's antiseptic system in 1867 was just the beginning of his work on putrefactive wounds. He continued to experiment with carbolic acid, which involved fine-tuning and making adjustments in his methods. Indeed, Lister's students—who might attend a demonstration with their minds settled on one technique, only to discover that their professor had already developed a new method since their last encounter—came to expect these changes. For them, it underlined the value of experimentation in medicine and illustrated that observational acuity and accuracy could lead to improvements in surgery.

From the beginning, Lister had advocated the wholesale sterilization with carbolic acid of everything from the instruments to the surgeon's hands, a protocol that led to the corrosion of his own skin over time. But ligatures—which were essential for tying off blood vessels during amputations or cutting off the blood supply in aneurysms—remained problematic even after he began dousing them with carbolic acid. It was customary to tie ligatures tightly and leave one or both ends of the knot long enough to protrude from the wound. Surgeons did this partly to allow for drainage and partly to make it easier to remove the ligature once the wound had healed. Unfortunately, this method also provided an easy path for contaminants.

Lister reasoned that if he could eliminate infection, there would be no drainage, and thus no need for ligatures to hang outside the wound. What he needed was a strong, flexible material that could be easily knotted, remain intact until its purpose had been fulfilled, and either become inactive or somehow be absorbed by the body. At first, Lister chose silk soaked in carbolic acid because its smooth surface was unlikely to irritate tissues. He sliced open the neck of a horse and tied off the major artery using a silk ligature. Six weeks later, the horse died unexpectedly of an unrelated cause. Lister was in bed with a cold at the time, and so he asked his assistant Hector Cameron to dissect out the left side of the horse's neck and report to his home later that day. At 11:00 p.m., Cameron brought the specimen to the ailing surgeon, who forced himself out of bed and worked until the early hours of the morning to isolate the ligated site. It was as he had predicted: the silk remained but was now encapsulated in fibrous tissue.

The opportunity soon presented itself for Lister to test the silk ligatures on a human patient. A woman had come to him suffering from an aneurysm in the leg. Lister soaked the silk in carbolic acid before using it to tie off the artery that was feeding the swelling. The patient survived, only to die ten months later when a second aneurysm ruptured. Lister obtained the dead body and performed a postmortem examination. He discovered that the silk ligature had been absorbed; however, there was a tiny pocket of pus near the opening, which he worried was the beginning of an abscess. Clearly, silk ligatures were not going to be the long-term solution he had hoped. So Lister turned his attention to another organic material: catgut.

The term "catgut" is something of a misnomer. The type of cord is actually prepared from the intestines of sheep or goat, although sometimes it can be made from the innards of cattle, hogs, horses, mules, or donkeys. Once again, Lister tested the ligature on an animal before moving on to humans, this time choosing a calf. His nephew Rickman John Godlee assisted Lister in the experiment: "I have a vivid recollection of the operation . . . the shaving and the purification of the part, the meticulous attention to every antiseptic detail, the dressing formed of a towel soaked in carbolic oil; and my grandfather's alabaster Buddha on the mantelpiece contemplating with inscrutable gaze the services of beast to man." A month later, the calf was slaughtered, the meat divided up among Lister's assistants, and the artery examined. The catgut ligature had been entirely absorbed by surrounding tissue.

Unfortunately, when Lister began testing the catgut on humans, he discovered that the material was absorbed so readily that it put the patient at risk of secondary hemorrhaging. He experimented with a wide variety of carbolic acid solutions and was able to slow the process down. After he published his report in *The Lancet*, the journal's editors commented that catgut ligature promised to be "far more than a mere contribution to practical surgery" because it demonstrated how dead organic material could be absorbed into a living body. Catgut quickly became a standard part of Lister's antiseptic treatment and was one example of the many ways in which his system evolved during these formative years.

Indeed, his obsession with improving the catgut ligatures spanned his entire career. After he moved to Edinburgh, he began meticulously recording notes from his experiments in three-hundred-page folio-sized notebooks, of which there were four by the time he retired. The very first entry in the first of these notebooks was about catgut, dated January 27, 1870. And the research notes conclude on the same subject in 1899.

As Lister's methods evolved, skeptics characterized these constant modifications as admissions on his part that the original system did not work. They didn't see these adjustments as part of the natural progression of a scientific process. James Y. Simpson waded back into the controversy, suggesting an almost fatalistic approach to the problem plaguing the country's hospitals. If cross-contamination could not be controlled, he argued, then hospitals should be periodically destroyed and built anew. Even Lister's old instructor John Eric Erichsen adopted this view. "Once a hospital has become incurably pyemia-stricken, it is impossible to disinfect it by any known hygienic means, as it would to disinfect an old cheese of the maggots which have been generated in it," he wrote. There was only one solution in Erichsen's mind, and it wasn't his former pupil's antiseptic system. He advocated the wholesale "demolition of the infected fabric."

But for all the opposition Lister faced, he was fighting the battle with like-minded people who recognized the revolutionary nature of his work. Initially, his antiseptic system received more support on the Continent than it did in Britain, so much so that in 1870 Lister was asked by both the French and the Germans to furnish some guide-lines for treating wounded soldiers fighting in the Franco-Prussian War. As a consequence, the German physician Richard von Volkmann became a spirited devotee after his hospital at Halle—overcrowded with wounded soldiers from the war and so dreadfully overcome with infection that its closure was imminent—achieved astonishing results by employing Lister's methods. Following this, Lister's system was taken up by other European surgeons, including a Dane named M. H. Saxtorph, who reported success in a letter to Lister. Armed with this testimony, Lister goaded the surgeons in London who had been the most critical of his antiseptic treatment: "It may seem strange that results like these should have been ob-tained in Copenhagen, when so little approach to them has yet been made in the capital of England."

Slowly but surely, surgeons in his own country began to rise in his defense. One of these men was Thomas Keith, a pioneer in ovariotomy, which was a dangerous procedure that involved the excision of ovarian tumors within the abdominal cavity. For most of the nineteenth century, ovariotomy remained extremely controversial. Those who dared to undertake such an invasive procedure were nicknamed "belly-rippers" on account of the long incision they made across the abdomen of their patients, which frequently became a source of sepsis.

Keith defended Lister against earlier attacks by Donald Campbell Black, who had not only dismissed Lister's work as the latest toy in medical science but also invoked Keith's name in his criticism of the antiseptic system. Keith replied to Black in the *British Medical Journal*. Contrary to what Black had implied, Keith *had* been dressing wounds "exactly as I have seen Mr. Lister do" and with great success. He was dismayed by the fact that Black, himself a surgeon from Glasgow, would attack a colleague when Lister had raised the reputation of the medical school in the city and given it a name. In his opinion, the antiseptic system was the future: "I think I am only now beginning to realise what Mr. Lister's antiseptic method and his carbolised animal-ligatures are yet to do for surgery." E. R. Bickersteth, a surgeon at the Royal Infirmary in Liverpool, also reported numerous cases in which he had effectively employed antiseptic catgut ligatures. He considered the antiseptic method "an immense step towards the perfection of our art."

By this time, Lister had already responded to charges that mortality rates hadn't decreased at the Glasgow Royal Infirmary after he introduced his antiseptic treatment. He compared the number of deaths on his wards from 1864 and 1866 with those from 1867 and 1868, after he began using carbolic acid. What he found was that sixteen of the thirty-five people who had undergone amputations had died prior to his introduction of his antiseptic treatment in 1864 and 1866, compared with only six of forty in the later years.

The report prompted the editor of *The Lancet* to call on hospitals in London to test Lister's antiseptic methods "fairly and crucially" a second time. He suggested that Lister's own students oversee the experiments. What had been achieved in Glasgow "ought to be procurable in London," the editor at the journal concluded. And so, in 1870, all eyes turned to the capital.

—

BACK IN EDINBURGH, John Rudd Leeson had only recently qualified as a surgeon when he approached the home of Joseph Lister. The man was visibly nervous. The house itself was "like a moat which made Lister still more inaccessible" than he already seemed to Leeson as he climbed the broad steps to the front door. He had come to ask the renowned professor if he could put his name on a wait list to become one of his surgical dressers at the hospital. Although Leeson had attended Lister's wards, he had yet to speak directly to the man whom he had come to admire so much.

The butler—a stern man whose demeanor had earned him the nickname "Mr. Bludgeon"—ushered Leeson into the private study where Lister was sitting before shutting the door behind him. The young surgeon found himself in a stately room dominated by glass-fronted mahogany bookcases and large north-facing windows. Lister stood up from behind his desk to greet Leeson, who "felt instinctively that I was in the presence of . . . the embodiment of high purpose." The elder surgeon put the novice at ease with what Leeson described as a "delightful and charming smile." After a brief conversation, Lister reached for a small ledger from one of the drawers in his desk and entered the man's name in its pages. He told Leeson that he could commence work as his surgical dresser the next winter.

As Leeson turned to leave, he noticed something odd on a table in front of the windows. Glittering in the sunlight and covered with glass shades were several rows of test tubes, half full of various liquids and plugged with cotton wool: Lister's Glass Garden. "It was a curious assemblage such as I had never seen, nor could I form the least conjecture as to what they were or why they should be plugged with cotton," he later wrote. "My experience of test-tubes was an open mouth and I never remember having seen them closed."

Seeing a sudden interest in the young surgeon's face, Lister rushed to his side, delighted to show Leeson his odd collection of liquids. He pointed out that some were turbid and moldy while others remained clear. "I tried to show an intelligent interest," Leeson confessed, "but had not the faintest idea as to what it was all about." As the professor pontificated about his most recent experiments into the causes of putrefaction, Leeson marveled that the renowned surgeon should have time to pursue such irrelevant and out-of-the-way matters.

Hoping to end the encounter on a high note, Leeson cast around for a subject on which he could speak coherently. That was when his eyes fell upon the large Powell and Lealand microscope sitting on Lister's desk. He told the professor that the revered octogenarian demonstrator at St. Thomas' Hospital in London who had taught him anatomy had used a similar instrument. Lister's eyes sparkled with excitement: mentioning the microscope "seemed to bring [him] back to reality." He chatted eagerly with Leeson about the importance of the instrument for the future of surgery.

"I had not the least idea that [the microscope] had any connection with the plugged test-tubes," Leeson later admitted. Although he had spent two and a half years at one of London's largest and most progressive hospitals, the newly qualified surgeon said that he had "never heard anything about microbes . . . and certainly had not the slightest idea that they had connection with medicine or surgery." The role of scientific knowledge and methodology in medical practice—which was central to the transition of the profession from a butchering art to a forward-looking discipline—had not yet been established. But the tide was turning in Lister's favor.

11.

THE QUEEN'S ABSCESS

—

Truth from his lips prevailed with double sway,

And fools, who came to scoff, remained to pray.

—OLIVER GOLDSMITH

LISTER'S CARRIAGE PULLED UP at the grand entrance of Balmoral Castle, the heart of Queen Victoria's sprawling estate in the Highlands of Scotland, on September 4, 1871. The day before, he had received an urgent telegraph requesting his presence at this royal residence. The queen was gravely ill. An abscess in her armpit had grown to the size of an orange, already measuring six inches in diameter. With Syme dead, Lister was now the most renowned surgeon in Scotland, so it was only natural that he would be consulted on a serious matter involving the queen's health.

Victoria's troubles had begun a few weeks earlier, when she developed a sore throat. Soon after, she experienced pain and swelling in her right arm. In a diary entry a short while later, the queen bemoaned the fact that her "arm [is] no better, & will not yield to any treatment. Every kind of thing has been tried." Her physicians begged the queen to allow a surgeon to be brought in. Not recognizing the severity of the situation, she demurred, but promised to think the matter over. Several days later, as the pain reached an excruciating level, Victoria finally consented.

The scrupulous surgeon carried everything with him that he would need to operate, including his latest invention: the carbolic spray. The idea for the apparatus had come to Lister a few months earlier and was, in part, prompted by a series of experiments carried out by the British physicist John Tyndall. By passing a concentrated ray of light through the air, Tyndall demonstrated the high content of dust floating in the atmosphere. He noticed that when the air was free from particles, however, the light disappeared. Tyndall rendered a sample of air dust-free with the use of heat and showed that putrescible solutions exposed to it remained sterile, while contact with air containing dust was soon corrupted by bacteria and mold. He spoke in amazement of the number of particles in the air "churning . . . in our lungs every hour and minute of our lives" and expressed concern over the effects they might have on surgical instruments in particular. For Lister, this merely reinforced the idea that germs in the air needed to be destroyed in medical environments. The carbolic spray was therefore designed to sterilize the air around the patient, both during an operation and afterward when changing dressings. But it had another purpose as well. Lister believed that the spray would reduce the need for direct irrigation of the wound with carbolic acid, which often damaged the skin and increased the risk of inflammation and infection.

At first, the apparatus was a handheld device, but like all of Lister's innovations it underwent several alterations during his lifetime. In one of its later forms—dubbed the "donkey engine"—a large copper atomizer sat on a tripod about three feet high. There was a foot-long handle on the atomizer that could be used to direct the spray. The entire mechanism weighed nearly ten pounds and was a cumbersome instrument that needed to be carried in with the help of Lister's assistants, who each took a turn working the apparatus during long hours in the operating theater. One of Lister's former students wrote that the "citizens of Edinburgh grew used to the sight of [him] driving through the streets, uncomfortably sharing the accommodation in his brougham with this formidable engine of his warfare."

As comical as the mechanism was, the use of carbolic spray was a significant moment in medical history. Before then, critics could point to Lister's treatment as an extension of traditional methods that involved cleaning wounds with some form of an antiseptic. The atomizer, however, signaled Lister's commitment to the germ theory, specifically the one put forward by Louis Pasteur. At this point, little work had been done in the way of differentiating one kind of bacterium from another, much less distinguishing between pathogenic and harmless bacteria. It was only decades later that Lister abandoned the carbolic spray when the German physician and microbiologist Robert Koch developed a technique for staining and growing bacteria in a Petri dish (named after his assistant Julius Petri). This enabled Koch to match particular microorganisms to specific diseases and advance the theory that bacteria exist as distinct species, each producing a unique clinical syndrome. Using his method, Koch showed that airborne pathogens were not the main culprit of wound infection, which meant that sterilizing the air was futile.

In 1871, however, Lister was very much committed to the technique, and so he brought the carbolic spray with him when he was called to the bedside of the queen. As Lister entered Victoria's grand bedchamber in Balmoral Castle, he was confident that his antiseptic system saved lives. Still, using carbolic acid on hospital patients, or even his own sister, was very different from using it to treat a queen. His reputation would be ruined if his actions caused lasting harm to the monarch. Lister must have felt considerable trepidation when he examined Victoria and recognized that the situation was now critical. If the abscess grew worse, any number of septic conditions might set in, and the queen could die.

Victoria reluctantly gave her permission for the operation to proceed. Writing in her diary later, she confessed, "I felt dreadfully nervous, as I bear pain so badly. I shall be given chloroform, but not very much, as I am so far from well." In fact, she would remain semi-alert throughout the operation because Lister decided not to administer a heavy dose of the anesthetic on account of the queen's perilous state of health.

Lister called upon the help of the royal physician, William Jenner, whom he entrusted with the task of operating the carbolic spray during the procedure. As Lister began disinfecting his instruments, his hands, and the affected area under the queen's arm, Jenner pumped mists of carbolic acid into the air, filling the room with its distinctive aroma of sweet tar. When he was satisfied that sufficient quantities of the antiseptic were saturating the immediate area, Lister made a deep incision into Victoria's abscess. Blood and pus gushed from the wound. Lister carefully cleansed the cut, while Jenner continued with his energetic pumping of carbolic acid, covering everyone in the vicinity with white clouds of the corrosive substance. At one point, the royal physician fumbled with the awkward contraption and accidentally sprayed the queen in the face. When she complained, Jenner half jokingly replied that he was only the man who worked the bellows. Once the procedure was over, Lister carefully bandaged the wound and left the exhausted monarch to rest.

The next day, as Lister was changing Victoria's dressings, he noticed that pus had formed underneath the linen that he had placed over the surgical wound. Lister needed to act quickly to prevent infection from setting in. Spying the atomizer, he had an idea. He took the rubber tubing off the apparatus, soaked it overnight in carbolic acid, and inserted it into the wound the following morning in order to drain the pus. The following day, Lister's nephew wrote that his uncle "rejoiced to find nothing escape [from the wound] unless it were a drop or so of clear serum." Lister himself later claimed that this was the first time he used such a drain. His ingenious ad hoc invention, along with his application of antiseptic methods, undoubtedly saved Victoria's life. One week later, Lister left Balmoral Castle and returned to Edinburgh, satisfied with the queen's recovery.

Back in the classroom, he quipped to his students, "Gentlemen, I am the only man who has ever stuck a knife into the Queen!"

News of Joseph Lister's successful treatment of Victoria spread, bolstering faith in his methods. The queen had given Lister's antiseptic system the royal stamp of approval simply by allowing him to operate on her. Furthermore, James Y. Simpson had died from a heart condition, putting an end to the feud that had blighted Lister's work for several years.

Shortly after Lister's encounter with royalty, Louis Pasteur traveled to London. On that trip, John Tyndall—who had recently visited Lister's wards in Glasgow—casually mentioned to the French scientist that "a celebrated English surgeon" had made an important contribution toward understanding the causes of putrid and contagious diseases using Pasteur's work as a guide. This was the first time Pasteur had ever heard of Lister. His interest was piqued.

The two men began a lengthy correspondence. In their letters, they discussed their experiments, theories, and discoveries and expressed mutual respect and esteem. Lister saw Pasteur as the man who had provided the means by which he could understand wound sepsis. In turn, Pasteur was in awe of Lister's advancement of the subject. As Pasteur wrote, "I am extremely surprised at the precision of your manipulations, [and] at your perfect comprehension of the experimental method." He was amazed that Lister could find the time to conduct such complex research while also attending to his patients. "It is a perfect enigma to me," he wrote to Lister, "that you can devote yourself to researches which demand so much care, time and incessant painstaking, at the same time as you devote yourself to the profession of surgery and to that of chief surgeon to a great hospital. I do not think that another instance of such a prodigy could be found amongst us here." To Lister—a man who had always placed immense faith in the scientific method—this was as high a compliment as could be paid him, especially since it came from such a revered figure as Pasteur.

As his own fame spread, Lister's classrooms swelled with students and eminent visitors from all over the world who had come to Edinburgh to witness the surgeon in action. He traveled around the country, expounding the virtues of his antiseptic system to medical audiences. And heartening reports finally began to emerge from London. *The Lancet*'s call to action had worked: hospitals in the capital were once again testing the efficacy of the antiseptic system. This time, the results were more encouraging than they had been at the end of the 1860s, shortly after Lister first published his findings. St. George's Hospital announced a rise in confidence in Lister's methods among its staff. Middlesex Hospital expressed similar sentiments after attaining positive results with both carbolic acid and zinc chloride. But the strongest support came from London Hospital, where nearly fifty surgical procedures performed in the past year were "conspicuous for the small amount of constitutional disturbance produced by very severe injuries" after surgeons began employing the antiseptic system.

Although there had been a perceptible shift in opinion toward the acceptance of Lister's methods in the capital, it took several more years before the wholesale adoption of antisepsis occurred in London. This was largely due to the fact that many surgeons in the city were unwilling to endorse Pasteur's germ theory of putrefaction. One London surgeon mocked Lister and his pioneering work by closing the door of his operating theater with a loud bang in order to "shut out Mr. Lister's germs." In a letter that appeared in *The Lancet*, a correspondent who signed his name "Flaneur" made a perceptive observation regarding the city's slow adoption of antisepsis:

> The truth is, that this is a question in science rather than in surgery, and hence, while eagerly adopted by the scientific Germans, and a little grudgingly by the semi-scientific Scotch, the antiseptic doctrine has never been in any degree appreciated or understood by the plodding and practical English surgeon. Happily for his patients, he has for a long time been to a considerable extent practising a partially antiseptic system, thanks to his cleanly English instincts; but it has been like the lady who talked prose without knowing it.

It was easier for Lister to convince doctors in Glasgow and Edinburgh of the value of his antiseptic system because each of those cities had one hospital and one university at its heart. London's medical community was far more fragmented and less scientifically minded. Clinical teaching was not yet as common in the capital as it was in Scotland. Lister railed, "If I turn to London, and ask how instruction in clinical surgery is conducted there, I find that not only according to my own experience as a London student . . . but also from the universal testimony of foreigners who visit there and then come here, it is, when compared with our system here, a mere sham." These were obstacles Lister could not overcome unless he could reform the system from within.

There was one group who never doubted Lister's antiseptic treatment: the people who survived because of it. An elderly man who had been admitted to the hospital both before and after Lister had introduced his system onto the wards remarked on the differences he saw: "Man, but ye hae made a grand improvement since I was here afore." Even those outside the profession who had not been Lister's patients were getting wind of miraculous recoveries. In a letter to her sister-in-law, Agnes Lister recounted the story of a boy whose life had been saved with carbolic acid after he had been severely burned while working in a local foundry. Patrick Heron Watson—who was once Lister's house surgeon—met with the Listers on the day of the accident. He told the couple that "*he did not think that* the boy could recover," Agnes wrote, "but by the help of carbolic acid, he *is* recovering and the case has excited great interest in several foundries." In fact, deputations of workmen came to the hospital to see the boy for themselves. Agnes wrote that "the boy's masters will appoint Dr. Watson surgeon to their works which will give him a salary of £300 a year" as a result. Another house surgeon who worked with Lister later wrote, "If recognition on the part of his colleagues was slow in coming, patients who had had experience under both systems, the old and the new, were quick to perceive the difference."

Lister's fame abroad was underscored in 1875, during a much-feted European tour he undertook with Agnes to showcase his methods. Wards adhering to his system were celebrated by many for their "fresh, healthy atmosphere" and an "absence of any smell," while *The*

Lancet characterized his progress through the university towns of Germany, where his system was particularly popular, as a triumphal march. Still, one nation remained unconvinced of the merits of Lister's methods: the United States.

In fact, in several American hospitals, Lister's techniques had been banned; many doctors saw them as unnecessary and overly complicated distractions because they had not yet accepted the germ theory of putrefaction. Even by the mid-1870s, understanding of wound care and infection had barely progressed, despite Lister's theories and techniques appearing in American medical journals. The medical community had, for the most part, rejected his antiseptic methods as quackery. Transatlantic skepticism notwithstanding, in 1876 Joseph Lister turned his eyes west when he was invited to defend his methods at the International Medical Congress in Philadelphia. To bring about a change in American attitudes, Lister knew he would need to evangelize for his work in person. As it turned out, convincing the Americans of the merits of antisepsis would not be as straightforward as he hoped.

Five years after operating on the queen, Lister was ready to face his critics in America. In July 1876, he boarded the SS *Scythia*—the last of the famous Cunarders with full sail and steam capabilities—for its voyage from Liverpool to New York. The run normally took ten days, but the vessel was struck by a ferocious squall that splintered the mast of its main topsail, delaying the ship several days. It was the first of many hindrances the surgeon would face on his American journey.

Lister stepped off the train from New York to Philadelphia on September 3. Although he was not a vain man, the forty-nine-year-old surgeon still adhered to the prevailing fashion of the day: he parted his wavy hair to the side and sported meticulously groomed muttonchops, now tinged with gray. Dressed conservatively in his fitted waistcoat and high starched collar, he adjusted his outer clothing and took in his surroundings. There was a tangible atmosphere of excitement, as the city was swelling with crowds who had come to visit the Philadelphia Centennial Exhibition.

Lister was met on the platform by hawkers selling small umbrellas designed to protect their users from both the harsh sun and the occasional thunderstorms that bedeviled the city at that time of year. These devices could be mounted atop a gentleman's hat and adjusted by means of tapes attached to the shoulders. There were also hand-held fans, refreshing "arctic" drinks, and cups of ice for sale. Boys dressed in cutaway jackets and floppy bow ties touted guidebooks for a nickel apiece to new arrivals who would soon wander around with mouths agape at the extraordinary spectacle of the exhibition set out before them.

It had been a hundred years since the Declaration of Independence had been signed in Philadelphia, and the city was bursting with patriotic pride in celebration of the centenary. The Centennial Exhibition was designed to mark America's ascendancy as a leader in science and industry. In an era of large-scale fairs celebrating science and progress, the gathering in Philadelphia was even grander than London's Great Exhibition of 1851, which Lister visited with his father. It featured thirty thousand displays from thirty-seven nations of the world, spread over an impressive 450 acres of land. Zigzagging through the fairgrounds were eighty miles of asphalt, bubbling and melting in the unrelenting heat. The world's first monorail shuttled passengers the 150 yards between Horticultural Hall and Agricultural Hall. Sightseers gawped at an astonishing collection of exotic animals, including a fifteen-foot walrus, a polar bear, and a shark, all displayed alongside the weapons used to hunt them.

The focal point of the fair was Machinery Hall, where visitors could marvel at the engineering wonders of the age. Electric lights and elevators were powered by a 1,400-horsepower Corliss steam engine—the largest ever of its kind, weighing in at 650 tons. There were locomotives, fire trucks, printing presses, hulks of mining equipment, and magic lanterns. Recent innovations, such as the typewriter, a mechanical calculator, and Alexander Graham Bell's telephone, were debuted to the appreciative public.

By September, the Exhibition was averaging an astonishing 100,000 visitors a day. But the British surgeon who had traveled over four thousand miles of ocean to America had only one aim in mind: to prove the merits of his antiseptic system. As Lister picked his way through the crowds, he braced himself for what might be awaiting him at the International Medical Congress.

Lister's invitation to speak at the conference had come from one of his most vocal critics across the Atlantic. Samuel D. Gross was one of the country's preeminent surgeons and was also a nonbeliever in the existence of germs. The American surgeon was so set against Lister's antiseptic system that he had commissioned a painting a year earlier to celebrate his faith in the surgical status quo. In the *Portrait of Samuel D. Gross* (later known as *The Gross Clinic*), the artist Thomas Eakins depicts a dark and dingy operating theater. Gross, at the center of the scene, is operating on a boy who is suffering from osteomyelitis of the femur. The surgeon is surrounded by his assistants, one of whom probes the patient's wound with bloodied fingers. In the foreground, unsterilized instruments and bandages are displayed within reach of equally unclean hands. There is no sign that Lister's antiseptic methods are being used.

Some American surgeons had adopted Lister's antiseptic system, though they very much remained in the minority. For instance, George Derby—who would later become professor of hygiene at Harvard University—read about Lister's work shortly after it first appeared in *The Lancet*. Several weeks later, a nine-year-old boy who was suffering from a compound fracture of the middle thigh found himself in Derby's care. Derby set the leg and then used carbolic acid to dress the wound. He reported, "At the end of four weeks, the [carbolic-acid-soaked dressing] was removed, disclosing a round, superficial ulcer, half an inch in diameter, which in a couple of days was covered with a firm scab. There is now . . . firm union of the bone." Derby discussed his findings at a meeting of the Boston Society for Medical Improvement and published his observations in *The Boston Medical and Surgical Journal* on October 31 of that same year, crediting "Mr. Lyster [*sic*], a surgeon of Glasgow," as his source of inspiration.

Similarly, at Massachusetts General Hospital, George Gay treated three patients suffering from compound fractures with carbolic acid. "The wounds," explained Gay, "were treated essentially according to the method of Mr. Liston [*sic*]." The surgeon argued that the carbolic acid's antiseptic qualities were possessed by no other compound that he had encountered in his research. Gay had full faith in Lister's methods, as did two other surgeons at the hospital who used carbolic acid on at least five other patients during that period. Of course, a man changing the course of history is never without his detractors. The head surgeon, Henry Jacob Bigelow—a censorious and dogmatic man who was present at the historic operation with ether at Massachusetts General Hospital in 1846—banned Lister's antiseptic system shortly after Gay and his colleagues began using carbolic acid, calling it "medical hocus-pocus." He went as far as to threaten to fire those who ignored his orders.

With the paint barely dry on the depiction of traditional surgery that Samuel D. Gross had commissioned, Lister found himself in hostile territory. This was in spite of the fact that America had recently endured a civil war that claimed tens of thousands of lives due to the mismanagement of appalling battle injuries. For the duration of the war, American surgery remained crude, and wound infections spread unchecked. The bullet-riddled arms and legs of more than thirty thousand Union soldiers were amputated by battlefield surgeons, many of whom had little or no experience of treating trauma patients. Knives and saws were wiped free of gore with nothing more than dirty rags, if at all. Surgeons never washed their hands and were often covered in the blood and guts of previous patients at the commencement of a new operation. When linen and cotton were scarce, army surgeons used cold, damp earth to pack open wounds. When these wounds inevitably began to suppurate, they were praised for their laudable pus. Many surgeons had never even witnessed a major amputation or treated gunshot wounds when they joined their regiments, much to the detriment of those who fell under their care.

As horrific as the war was, doctors and surgeons gained a profound knowledge of clinical experience from treating seemingly numberless battlefield casualties, which in turn accelerated surgical specialization in American medicine. Most important, they acquired administrative skills that enabled them to organize ambulance corps and commission hospital trains. Soon after the war was over, veteran surgeons began to design, staff, and manage vast general hospitals. This made their profession more cohesive in its operational procedures and made it ripe for a new approach to the art of surgery when Lister arrived in the country.

At noon on September 4, Lister entered the University of Pennsylvania's ornate chapel with other attendees of the International Medical Congress. On this first day, the antiseptic system came under immediate assault, with Lister sitting in the front row as speaker after speaker stood up to denounce all he believed in. One physician from New York noted that there was no satisfactory proof that germs were necessarily connected to illnesses such as cholera, diphtheria, erysipelas, or any other infectious disease. Another doctor, from Canada, cautioned, "Is it not to be feared that the particular treatment advised by Prof. Lister tends to divert the attention of the surgeon from other essential points?" The final blow came from Frank Hamilton, a battle-hardened Civil War hero, who reproached Lister directly. "A large portion of American surgeons seem not to have adopted your practice," he said, looking down at the British surgeon from his podium; "whether from a lack of confidence or for other reasons, I cannot say."

When the diatribes against him had at last ended, all eyes turned to this divisive figure. But Lister would have to wait till the second day of the conference to address his opponents. At the allotted hour on that day, he made his way to the front of the chapel, and he readied himself to defend a system he was certain could save tens of thousands dying in hospitals at that very moment. He flattered his audience: "American physicians are renowned throughout the world for their inventive genius, and boldness and skill in execution." It was to *their* credit that anesthesia was now used in surgery. For two and a half hours, Lister lectured on the merits of antisepsis, concentrating on the interrelationship between dirt, germs, pus, and wounds. He peppered his talk with entertaining demonstrations and case histories. His conclusions were shrewdly simple: if germs were destroyed during an operation and prevented from accessing a wound afterward, no pus would form. "The germ theory of putrefaction is the foundation of the whole system of antisepsis," Lister told his audience, "and, if this theory is a fact, it is a fact of facts that the antiseptic system means the exclusion of all putrefactive organisms."

If Lister had nursed any hope that his diligence and reasoned argument concerning his antiseptic system would convert the American audience, he would be sorely disappointed. One attendee accused him of being mentally unhinged and having a "grasshopper in the head." Others berated him for speaking so long. "The hour being late," one critic whined, "I merely desire to point out a few facts which . . . militate against the [germ] theory, as far as it claims that a certain class of minute living organisms . . . are essential to disease-processes." But it was Samuel Gross—the man who had hoped to discredit Lister by inviting him to speak at the International Medical Congress—who would have the final word: "Little, if any faith, is placed by any enlightened or experienced surgeon on this side of the Atlantic in the so-called treatment of Professor Lister."

Lister would not be easily deterred from winning over American hearts and minds to his antiseptic system. After the conference, he set out on a transcontinental train journey that took him as far as San Francisco and back. He stopped in several cities along the way, lecturing to crowded rooms of medical students and surgeons about the value of antisepsis. Many of these men went on to test the efficacy of his system on their own patients and reported positive results.

In Chicago, Lister's host was a former patient whom he had treated in Glasgow after she was injured in a mill. Although the woman had made a good recovery, she was no longer capable of manual labor after the accident. Concerned about her future, Lister intervened with the woman's employer and asked that she be given a trial working in the department for design. She did so well at her new job that the firm sent her to America, where she was put in charge of the company's exhibit at another fair held in Chicago, several years before the one Lister had attended in Philadelphia. While there, she met a young American manufacturer and married. When she heard of Lister's visit, she was thrilled to welcome the man who had saved her life and open to him the doors of her home for the duration of his visit.

Toward the end of his trip, Lister performed an operation on Blackwell's Island (now Roosevelt Island) in New York City. He had come at the request of William Van Buren, a distinguished surgeon who had heard Lister speak in Philadelphia. It turned out there were a few attendees who privately supported Lister. For instance,

William W. Keen, a pioneer in neurological surgery, adopted antisepsis a month after the International Medical Congress. He later recounted, "For me it changed surgery from Purgatory to Paradise," adding that he would never abandon Lister's system. D. Hayes Agnew, also in attendance, adopted Lister's techniques as well. Shortly afterward, he highlighted the subject in his book *The Principles and Practice of Surgery.* And then there was Van Buren, who was so impressed by Lister's lecture that he invited him to perform a surgical demonstration for his students. On the appointed day, Lister watched in amazement as more than a hundred of Van Buren's students filled the auditorium of Charity Hospital. "I had no idea that I was to address so large a body of students," Lister said to the crowd. "It is a most unexpected privilege."

Lister prepared to demonstrate his antiseptic techniques on a young man who had developed a large syphilitic abscess on his groin. He began by dipping his instruments and his hands in a basin full of carbolic acid as the patient was administered chloroform. While preparations were under way, one of the spectators opened a window to let in some air because the operating theater was packed to capacity. A hush fell over the room. Lister directed a volunteer to pump carbolic acid into the air directly over the operating table. As he was about to make an incision, a slight breeze blew the solution away from the patient. Turning to the window, Lister asked that it be shut and then used the episode to caution those in attendance that rigorous attention to all the details of the antisepsis routine was mandatory. He proceeded to operate, carefully slicing open the infected abscess, draining it of infective pus, and irrigating the wound with carbolic acid before wrapping the groin and upper thigh in antiseptic bandages. Lister's lecture was recorded word for word by a student in the audience. When the demonstration was complete, the crowd cheered.

Before heading back to Britain, Lister moved on to Boston, and it would prove to be a serendipitous visit. There, he met Henry J.

Bigelow, the man who had banned his antiseptic techniques at Massachusetts General Hospital. Bigelow hadn't attended the medical conference in Philadelphia, but he had read reports about Lister's lecture. Although he still wasn't convinced about the existence of germs, he was impressed by Lister's dedication to his system and the care and attention he paid his patients. Bigelow invited Lister to speak at Harvard University, where he was warmly received by the medical students in attendance. Not long afterward, the American surgeon delivered a lecture of his own. In it, he praised "the new doctrine" and confessed his conversion to Lister's antiseptic system: "I have learned that the duty of the surgeon . . . should be to destroy the actual intruders [germs], and effectually to exclude their thronging companions."

With Bigelow's endorsement, Massachusetts General became the first hospital in America to make institutional use of carbolic acid as a surgical antiseptic. It was an extraordinary volte-face of policy in a hospital that for years had banned Lister's methods and even threatened to fire those who dared implement them.

Lister returned to Britain, reenergized by the more positive reactions by Americans to his antiseptic system toward the end of his trip. Not long after he had settled back into Edinburgh life in February 1877, Lister received news that the renowned Sir William Fergusson had died. He had been professor of surgery at King's College in London for thirty-seven years. After his death, the university approached Lister about the position. With the gradual acceptance of antisepsis at home and beyond Britain's shores, Lister's reputation was enviable. Students flocked to his classroom in record numbers. Prominent foreigners traveled thousands of miles to visit his wards and witness his operations. Although King's College could have promoted Fergusson's colleague John Wood, the members of the university's council were inclined to prefer someone more distin-guished to fill the vacancy. They could think of no one better suited to the role than Joseph Lister.

Unsurprisingly, Lister had concerns. He worried that he would not be given the same degree of freedom in London that he had been granted in Edinburgh and responded to the unofficial offer from the university's council members by laying out conditions of his own. He told them that if he were to take up the position at King's Col-lege, his aim would be to introduce and diffuse his antiseptic system throughout the capital. He also hoped to institute a more efficient method of clinical teaching at the university, with an emphasis on practical demonstrations and experimentation.

Back in Edinburgh, Lister's students were devastated when news about the negotiations and of his possible departure was leaked. At the end of one of his clinical lectures, they presented him with a formal plea signed by more than seven hundred students. Isaac Bayley Balfour, one of his pupils, read the document aloud: "We eagerly seize this occasion to acknowledge the deep debt of gratitude we owe the in-valuable instruction we have derived from your clinical teaching. . . . [M]any have gone forth, and many will still go forth, determined to carry your principles into practice and spread . . . that system of sur-gery of which you are the founder." The students applauded this sentiment. When the class had quieted down, Balfour continued. "The welfare of our school is so intimately bound up with your pres-ence," he told Lister, "we would yet earnestly hope that . . . the day may never come when your name will cease to be associated with that of the Edinburgh Medical School." Lister was overwhelmed by his students' response. To their delight, he told them that even if he should secure the topmost position in private practice in London, he could not take up a position at King's College if it meant teaching clinical surgery in the way it was currently being taught throughout the capital.

Both the students' address and Lister's response were subsequently reported in newspapers around the country. Word reached King's College that Lister had been vocally critical of prevailing teaching methods in London. Tempers flared. *The Lancet* reported that Lister had forgotten "the rules of decency and good taste as to contemptuously decline an offer that had never been made to him." And just a few weeks later, the governing council at King's College appointed John Wood to Fergusson's chair.

Lister's friends in London hadn't abandoned the fight just yet. Because there had been no formal offer made to him, there had also been no formal rejection. In April, a resolution was put before the council requesting that a second chair of clinical surgery be created and that Lister be considered for the position because "it would be a great benefit to the school." This time, cooler heads prevailed—much to the dismay of poor Wood, who did not relish the idea of sharing his role with another surgeon. In May, Lister traveled to London to meet with the council and presented them with *thirteen* conditions. Driving a hard bargain, he stipulated that he wished to retain total control over his wards and his classroom and that the division of fees between him and Wood should be fair. The council members reluctantly accepted his conditions because they knew that having such a renowned professor on their staff would elevate the reputation of the university. Shortly afterward, Lister was officially appointed professor of clinical surgery at King's College.

It was a bittersweet moment. For nearly a quarter of a century, Lister had hoped to return to London one day, and now at the age of fifty he had finally been granted that opportunity. But leaving Edinburgh at the height of his career and beginning anew would not be an easy undertaking. Decades earlier, it had been the material rewards and career advancement that had underpinned his desire to move back to the capital. This time, it was the London medical community's stubborn disbelief in his antiseptic system. His was a mission to convert the nonbelievers, just as he had done in Glasgow and Edinburgh, and throughout America.

In September 1877, Lister slipped quietly away from the Scottish city where he had first fallen in love with the bloodied and butchering art of surgery under the tutelage of his great mentor, James Syme. But just before boarding the train, he made a valedictory check upon his final intake of patients at the Royal Infirmary. As he walked the hallways one last time, he took stock of the institute's marked transformation. He was confident that it would be safe in the hands of his disciples, who would now be entrusted with implementing his antiseptic system throughout the hospital. Gone were the filthy wards crammed with patients wasting away in squalid conditions; gone were the bloodied aprons and the operating tables soiled with bodily fluids; and gone were the unwashed instruments, all of which once had the operating theater reeking of "good old hospital stink." The Royal Infirmary was now bright, clean, and well ventilated. No longer a house of death, it was a house of healing.

EPILOGUE:
THE DARK CURTAIN,
RAISED

—

**It is Surgery that, long after it has passed
into obsolescence, will be remembered
as the glory of Medicine.**

—RICHARD SELZER

IN DECEMBER 1892, JOSEPH LISTER traveled to Paris to attend a
grand celebration of Louis Pasteur's seventieth birthday. Hundreds
of delegates from around the world gathered at the Sorbonne to
pay homage to the scientist, and to express admiration on behalf of
their respective countries for the groundbreaking work he had conducted over the course of his career. Lister was present not just as a
representative of the Royal Societies of London and Edinburgh but
as Pasteur's friend and intellectual companion.

On that crisp winter day in Paris, the two men entered the Sorbonne, both preeminent exponents of their respective fields. In addition to foreign dignitaries, thousands of members of the public gathered to watch the celebration. Despite the jubilant atmosphere, however, not all was well privately. Both men were advancing in years, and life seemed to be winding down for the two of them. Lister, now sixty-five, had reached the age at which retirement from his professorship at King's College was compulsory. Within a few months, his wife and companion of thirty-seven years would die, leaving a void that would never be filled. Pasteur had recently suffered a stroke—the second of three that he would experience during his lifetime. Once, when writing to Lister back in London, Pasteur reflected on his suffering: "The impairment of my speech has become permanent, just as the partial paralysis of my left side has become permanent." On the day of the celebration, the intellectual giant hobbled onto the stage, unable to move effectively without assistance.

Lister paid tribute to the French scientist during his address. In his typically humble way, he downplayed his own role in the transformation of surgery. Instead, Lister credited Pasteur with "raising the dark curtain" in medicine. "You have changed Surgery . . . from being a hazardous lottery into a safe and soundly-based science," he said of Pasteur. "You are the leader of the modern generation of scientific surgeons, and every wise and good man in our profession—especially in Scotland—looks up to you with respect and attachment as few men receive." If the stroke hadn't severely hindered his ability to speak, Pasteur might have expressed exactly the same sentiments about Lister.

The auditorium erupted into thunderous applause as Lister concluded his tribute. Pasteur rose from his chair and with the help of attendants embraced his old friend. According to an official record of the occasion, it was "like the living picture of the brotherhood of science in the relief of humanity."

The two would never again meet in person.

—

LISTER LIVED FOR MANY DECADES after his theories and techniques had been accepted, and he was eventually celebrated as a hero of surgery. He was appointed personal surgeon in ordinary to Queen Victoria—the term "in ordinary" signaling that it was a permanent position. In the final decades of his life, official accolades came thick and fast. He was awarded honorary doctorates from the Universities of Cambridge and Oxford. He was awarded the Boudet Prize for the single greatest contribution to medicine. Shortly afterward, he attended the International Medical Congress in London. In contrast to his circumstances at the first of these gatherings, held in Philadelphia, Lister's reputation and methods had reached their acme by the time the medical community reconvened in the British capital. He was also knighted and made a baronet; he was elected president of the Royal Society; he was raised to the peerage and titled Lord Lister of Lyme Regis; he helped found the medical research body that would later be named in his honor, the Lister Institute of Preventive Medicine; and ten years before his death he was made privy councillor and honored with the Order of Merit—all for his work in science and medicine.

The burgeoning awareness of microbes intensified the Victorian public's preoccupation with cleanliness, and a new generation of carbolic acid cleaning and personal hygiene products flooded onto the market. Perhaps the most famous of these was Listerine, invented by Dr. Joseph Joshua Lawrence in 1879. Lawrence had attended Lister's lecture in Philadelphia, which inspired him to begin manufacturing his own antiseptic concoction in the back of an old cigar factory in

St. Louis shortly thereafter. Lawrence's formula contained thymol (derived from phenol) in addition to eucalyptol and menthol. It also had an alcohol concentration of 27 percent.

Nothing would have come of Listerine had the entrepreneurial pharmacist Jordan Wheat Lambert not recognized its potential when he met Lawrence in 1881. Lambert bought the rights to the product and its formula from the good doctor and began marketing it as an antiseptic with multiple uses, including as a dandruff treatment, a floor cleaner, and even a cure for gonorrhea. In 1895, Lambert promoted Listerine to the dental profession as an oral antiseptic, a use for which it has achieved immortality.

Other products that sprang up in the wake of the antiseptic mania included carbolic soap, carbolic general disinfectants (often simply neat phenol sold in bottles with instructions printed on them), and carbolic tooth powder. Calvert's Carbolic Tooth Paste became a household favorite and even attracted the patronage of Queen Victoria. In the United States, a practitioner in Illinois was the first to use carbolic acid for injecting into hemorrhoids, a dubious practice that more often than not left the recipient unable to walk for weeks. The wondrous properties of carbolic acid became so celebrated that a song was written about them. Clarence C. Wiley was a pharmacist from Iowa who won fame for his folk rag titled "Car-Balick-Acid Rag," composed and copyrighted in 1901. It was published as sheet music and in the form of a player piano roll.

There were hazards for the ill-informed: in September 1888, the *Aberdeen Evening Express* reported that thirteen people had been poisoned by carbolic acid in just one incident, and five of them had died. Later regulation in Britain prevented the sale of toxic chemicals in their purest form to the general public. Carbolic acid was also at the center of a corporate legal suit in 1892. The worryingly named Carbolic Smoke Ball was marketed in London as a prophylactic against influenza, in the wake of the flu pandemic that killed one million people between 1889 and 1890. The product was a rubber ball filled with carbolic acid and with a tube attached. This tube was to be inserted into the user's nose, and the ball was squeezed to release vapors. The nose would then run, the idea being that this would flush out infections.

As a marketing ploy that they assumed no buyer would take literally, the Smoke Ball's manufacturers advertised that those who found the product ineffective would be compensated with one hundred pounds—an extraordinary sum at the time. The judge presiding over a lawsuit that resulted from this error of judgment rejected the Carbolic Smoke Ball Company's claims that this was "mere puff" and ruled that the advertisement had made an unambiguous promise to customers. He ordered the company to pay compensation to an influenza sufferer and disappointed Smoke Ball purchaser named Louisa Carlill. To this day, the case is often cited to law students as an example of the basic principles of contractual obligation.

Among the more surprising offshoots of Lister's work was the establishment of one of the most recognizable corporations in the world today. Like the inventor of Listerine, Robert Wood Johnson first became aware of antisepsis when he attended Lister's lecture at the International Medical Congress in Philadelphia. Inspired by what he had heard that day, Johnson joined forces with his two brothers James and Edward, and founded a company to manufacture the first sterile surgical dressings and sutures mass-produced according to Lister's methods. They named it Johnson & Johnson.

But Lister's most enduring legacy was the successful and widespread dissemination of his ideas, attributable as much to a small but dedicated group of his students—the core Listerians—as to his own dogged persistence during those long years of controversy surrounding his antiseptic system. At the end of his career, Lister was often followed by a procession of solemn, reverential students, the first of whom bore aloft the sacred carbolic spray as a talisman of their mentor's extraordinary accomplishments. They came from all over the world to study under the great surgeon: from Paris, Vienna, Rome, and New York. And they took back with them his ideas, his methods, and his unshakable conviction that with the correct application of meticulous and hard-won techniques surgery could one day save far more lives than it inadvertently ended.

The adoption of Lister's antiseptic system was the most prominent outward sign of the medical community's acceptance of a germ theory, and it marked the epochal moment when medicine and science merged. Thomas Eakins—the artist who painted *The Gross Clinic*— returned to the subject in 1889 to paint *The Agnew Clinic*. This time, however, instead of painting a dingy operating theater with surgeons caked in blood, Eakins shows the viewer a markedly cleaner, brighter operating environment with participants wearing stark white coats. *The Agnew Clinic* portrays the embodiment of antisepsis and hygiene. It is Listerism, triumphant.

As the years passed, there was a gradual shift in medical procedure from antisepsis (germ killing) to asepsis (germ-free practices). The very theory on which Lister based his entire system seemed to demand that aseptic methods replace antisepsis. But he opposed this change because he felt asepsis—which required the scrupulous sterilization of everything within the patient's vicinity before procedures commenced—was impractical if surgeons were to continue operating outside the controlled environment of a hospital. Surgery, he felt, should be safe whether it was performed on one's dining table or in an operating theater, and antisepsis was the only viable solution when it came to operating in a patient's own home.

Lister recognized the importance of the hospital, but only in relation to the care and treatment of the poor. His former student Guy Theodore Wrench later argued that had it not been for his mentor's work, hospitals might have ceased to exist altogether. "Large hospitals were being abandoned and hut hospitals substituted," Wrench wrote.

"Lister's work . . . came in the nick of time. It saved not only patients but hospitals. It prevented . . . an entire reversion of the method of dealing surgically with the poor." But as essential as hospitals were, Lister did not think that the whole of his profession would be (or should be) based in them; those with means, he believed, would continue to be treated outside institutional walls, in their homes or in private clinics.

As he neared the end of his life, Lister expressed the desire that if his story was ever told, it would be done through his scientific achievements alone. In his will—dated June 26, 1908—the eighty-one-year-old surgeon requested that Rickman John Godlee, along with his other nephew Arthur Lister, "arrange [his] scientific manuscripts and sketches, destroying or otherwise disposing of such as are of no permanent scientific value or interest."

Lister wrongly believed that his personal story had little bearing on his scientific and surgical achievements. Ideas are never created in a vacuum, and Lister's life very much attests to that truth. From the moment he looked through the lens of his father's microscope to the day he was knighted by Queen Victoria, his life was shaped and influenced by his circumstances and the people around him. Like all of us, he saw his world through the prism of opinions held by those whom he admired most: Joseph Jackson, a supportive father and accomplished microscopist; William Sharpey, his instructor at UCL who encouraged him to go to Edinburgh; James Syme, his longtime mentor and father-in-law; and Louis Pasteur, the scientist who gave him the key needed to unlock one of the great medical mysteries of the nineteenth century.

Lister died peacefully on a cold, wintry morning in February 1912. Near his bedside were unfinished papers on the nature and causes of suppuration—a subject that had fascinated him since his student days. Even at the end, when his vision and hearing were severely impaired, Lister continued to engage with the scientific world around him. After his death, all his wishes were carried out, except one. His private and family correspondence was not destroyed, but preserved by his nephew. It is through his writing that we are first allowed a glimpse into Lister's inner sanctum.

Joseph Jackson had once reminded his son that it was a blessing that he had been permitted to be the means by which the antiseptic system was introduced to "thy fellow mortals." A life of self-sacrifice and singular determination had been fully vindicated. His pioneering work ensured that the results of surgery would no longer be left to chance. Henceforth, the ascendancy of knowledge over ignorance, and diligence over negligence, defined the profession's future. Surgeons became proactive rather than reactive when it came to postoperative infection. No longer lauded for their quick hand with a knife, they were revered for being careful, methodical, and precise. Lister's methods transformed surgery from a butchering art to a modern science, one where newly tried and tested methodologies trumped hackneyed practices. They opened up new frontiers in medicine—allowing us to delve further into the living body—and in the process they saved hundreds of thousands of lives.

Hector Cameron, Lister's former student and assistant, later said of him, "We *knew* we were in contact with Genius. We felt we were helping in the making of History and that all things were becoming new." What was once impossible was now achievable. What was once inconceivable could now be imagined. The future of medicine suddenly seemed limitless.

NOTES

PROLOGUE: THE AGE OF AGONY

3 *When a distinguished but elderly scientist*: Arthur C. Clarke, *Profiles of the Future* (London: Victor Gollancz Ltd, 1962), 25.

4 *The surgeon John Flint South*: John Flint South, *Memorials of John Flint South: Twice President of the Royal College of Surgeons, and Surgeon to St. Thomas's Hospital*, collected by the Reverend Charles Lett Feltoe (London: John Murray, 1884), 27.

4 *People were packed like herrings*: Ibid., 127, 128, 160.

4 *The audience was made up*: Ibid., 127.

4 *parts gushing forth not only*: Paolo Mascagni, *Anatomia universa XLIV* (Pisa: Capurro, 1823), quoted in Andrew Cunningham, *The Anatomist Anatomis'd: An Experimental Discipline in Enlightenment Europe* (Farnham, U.K.: Ashgate, 2010), 25.

4 *"What a terrible sight"*: Jean-Jacques Rousseau, "Seventh Walk," in *Reveries of the Solitary Walker*, trans. Peter France (Harmondsworth, U.K.: Penguin, 1979), 114, quoted in Cunningham, *Anatomist Anatomis'd*, 25.

5 *In 1840, for instance*: J. J. Rivlin, "Getting a Medical Qualification in England in the Nineteenth Century," http://www.evolve360.co.uk/data/10/docs/09/09rivlin.pdf, based on a paper delivered to a joint meeting of the Liverpool Medical History Society and the Liverpool Society for the History of Science and Technology, Oct. 12, 1996.

5 *"every thing that may incite terror"*: Thomas Percival, *Medical Jurisprudence; or a Code of Ethics and Institutes, Adapted to the Professions of Physic and Surgery* (Manchester, 1794), 16.

6 *"The actual mortality in hospitals"*: Florence Nightingale, *Notes on Hospitals*, 3rd ed. (London: Longman, Green, Longman, Roberts, and Green, 1863), iii.

7 *"We are going to try"*: Quoted in Peter Vinten-Johansen et al., *Cholera, Chloroform, and the Science of Medicine: A Life of John Snow* (Oxford: Oxford University Press, 2003), 111. See also Richard Hollingham, *Blood and Guts: A History of Surgery* (London: BBC Books, 2008); Victor Robinson, *Victory over Pain: A History of Anesthesia* (London: Sigma Books, 1947), 141–50; Alison Winter, *Mesmerized: Powers of the Mind in Victorian Britain* (Chicago: University of Chicago Press, 1998), 180.

7 *"quiets all suffering"*: Quoted in Steve Parker, *Kill or Cure: An Illustrated History of Medicine* (London: DK, 2013), 174.

8 *"It has long been"*: Henry Jacob Bigelow, "Insensibility During Surgical Operations Produced by Inhalation," *The Boston Medical and Surgical Journal*, Nov. 18, 1846, 309.

10 *At six feet two, Liston was*: Timothy J. Hatton, "How Have Europeans Grown So Tall?," *Oxford Economic Papers*, Sept. 1, 2013.

10 *"the gleam of his knife"*: D'A. Power, "Liston, Robert (1794–1847)," rev. Jean Loudon, *Oxford Dictionary of National Biography* (Oxford: Oxford University Press, 2004), www.oxforddnb.com.

11 *"Painful methods are always"*: John Pearson, *Principles of Surgery* (Boston: Stimpson & Clapp, 1832), vii.

11 *The traumas of the operating theater*: Myrtle Simpson, *Simpson the Obstetrician* (London: Victor Gollancz Ltd., 1972), 41, in A. J. Youngson, *The Scientific Revolution in Victorian Medicine* (London: Croom Helm, 1979), 28.

11 *The boy asked the surgeon*: F. W. Cock, "Anecdota Listoniensa," *University College Hospital Magazine* (1911): 55, quoted in Peter Stanley, *For Fear of Pain: British Surgery, 1790–1850* (New York: Rodopi, 2002), 313.

11 *Sixty years later, Pace would*: Pace is also mentioned by Liston in his casebooks. See Liston casebook, Dec. 1845–Feb. 1847, UCH/MR/1/61, University College London.

13 *"fat, plethoric, and with a liver"*: Quoted in Harold Ellis, *A History of Surgery* (London: Greenwich Medical Media, 2001), 85.

13 *At twenty-five minutes past two*: Quoted in Hollingham, *Blood and Guts*, 59–64.

14 *An observer in the audience*: F. W. Cock, "The First Operation Under Ether in Europe: The Story of Three Days," *University College Hospital Magazine* 1 (1911): 127–44.

14 *Earlier in the century*: Charles Bell, *Illustrations of the Great Operations of Surgery* (London: Longman, 1821), 62, quoted in Stanley, *For Fear of Pain*, 83.

15 *In 1823, Thomas Alcock*: Thomas Alcock, "An Essay on the Education and Duties of the General Practitioner in Medicine and Surgery," *Transactions of the Associated Apothecaries and Surgeon Apothecaries of England and Wales* (London: Society, 1823), 53, quoted in Stanley, *For Fear of Pain*, 83.

15 *His contemporary William Gibson*: William Gibson, *Institutes and Practice of Surgery* (Philadelphia: James Kay, Jun. & Brother, 1841), 504, quoted in Stanley, *For Fear of Pain*, 83.

16 *"announcing in enthusiastic terms"*: James Miller, *Surgical Experience of Chloroform* (Edinburgh: Sutherland & Knox, 1848), 7, quoted in Stanley, *For Fear of Pain*, 295.

16 *"The history of Medicine has presented"*: "Etherization in Surgery," *Exeter Flying Post*, June 24, 1847, 4.

16 *"Oh, what delight for every feeling"*: "The Good News from America,"

in John Saunders, ed., *People's Journal* (London: People's Journal Office, 1846–[1849?]), Jan. 9, 1847, 25.

16 *"so horrible and distressing"*: T. G. Wilson, *Victorian Doctor, Being the Life of Sir William Wilde* (London: Methuen, 1942), 90, quoted in Stanley, *For Fear of Pain*, 174.

16 *Nor would they feel*: South, *Memorials of John Flint South*, 36.

17 *Patients worldwide came to further dread*: Jerry L. Gaw, *"A Time to Heal": The Diffusion of Listerism in Victorian Britain* (Philadelphia: American Philosophical Society, 1999), 8.

1. THROUGH THE LENS

19 *"Let us not overlook"*: Herbert Spencer, *Education: Intellectual, Moral, and Physical* (New York: D. Appleton, 1861), 81–82.

20 *Once, he plucked a shrimp*: Quoted in Sir Rickman John Godlee, *Lord Lister*, 2nd ed. (London: Macmillan, 1918), 28.

20 *"The baby has been today"*: Isabella Lister to Joseph Jackson Lister, Oct. 21, 1827, MS 6963/6, Wellcome Library.

21 *On the first floor*: Richard B. Fisher, *Joseph Lister, 1827–1912* (London: MacDonald and Jane's, 1977), 23.

22 *Before 1848, no major hospital*: Fisher, *Joseph Lister*, 35.

22 *"shade another man"*: Joseph Lister to Isabella Lister, Feb. 21, 1841, MS 6967/17, Wellcome Library.

23 *"I got almost all the meat off"*: Quoted in Godlee, *Lord Lister*, 14.

23 *"It looks just as if"*: Ibid.

23 *His village of Upton*: Ibid., 12.

23 *"folding windows open to the garden"*: Ibid., 8.

23 *"ghastly heap of fermenting brickwork"*: John Ruskin, *The Crown of Wild Olive* (1866), 14, in Edward Tyas Cook and Alexander Wedderburn (eds.), *The Works of John Ruskin*, vol. 18 (Cambridge, U.K.: Cambridge University Press, 2010), 406.

24 *Death was a frequent visitor*: Descriptions of graveyards come from Edwin Chadwick, *Report on the Sanitary Conditions of the Labouring Population of Great Britain: A Supplementary Report on the Results of a Special Inquiry into the Practice of Interment in Towns* (London: Printed by Clowes for HMSO, 1843), 134.

24 *two men purportedly asphyxiated*: Story from Ruth Richardson, *Death, Dissection, and the Destitute* (London: Routledge & Kegan Paul, 1987), 60.

24 *For those living near these pits*: For further descriptions of Clement's Lane, see Sarah Wise, *The Italian Boy: Murder and Grave-Robbery in 1830s London* (London: Pimlico, 2005), 52.

25 *An entire underground army*: For more on this subject, see Steven Johnson, *The Ghost Map: The Story of London's Most Terrifying Epidemic—and How It Changed Science, Cities, and the Modern World* (New York: Riverhead, 2006), 7–9.

25 *The business conducted elsewhere*: For more, see Kellow Chesney, *The Victorian Underworld* (Newton Abbot: Readers Union Group, 1970), 15–19, 95–97.

26 *When the young doctor*: Letter from Peter Mark Roget to his sister Annette, December 29, 1800. Quoted in D. L. Emblen, *Peter Mark Roget: The Word and the Man* (London: Longman, 1970), 54.

26 *The university was part of this*: "The London College," *Times*, June 6, 1825.

27 *"The morality of London"*: *John Bull*, Feb. 14, 1825.

28 *At five feet ten inches*: Hatton, "How Have Europeans Grown So Tall?"

28 *"When I was admitted to the drawing-room"*: Hector Charles Cameron, *Joseph Lister: The Friend of Man* (London: William Heinemann Medical Books, 1948), 16.

28 *Lister was described*: Ibid., 16–18.

28 *"He lived in the world"*: Thomas Hodgkin, Remembrance of Lister's Youth, April 5, 1911, MS 6985/12, Wellcome Library.

29 *"man in straightened [sic] circumstances"*: Ibid.

29 *In his account books*: Cashbook, Oct.–Dec. 1846, MS 6981, Wellcome Library.

30 *Hodgkin, who was five years*: Louise Creighton, *Life and Letters of Thomas Hodgkin* (London: Longmans, Green, 1917), 12.

30 *"a very suitable companion"*: Ibid., 39.

30 *"snares which notoriously lie"*: John Stevenson Bushnan, *Address to the Medical Students of London: Session 1850–1* (London: J. Churchill, 1850), 11, 12.

31 *"by-word for vulgar riot"*: William Augustus Guy, *On Medical Education* (London: Henry Renshaw, 1846), 23, quoted in Stanley, *For Fear of Pain*, 167.

31 *"apt to be lawless, exuberant"*: "Medical Education in New York," *Harper's New Monthly Magazine*, Sept. 1882, 672, quoted in Michael Sappol, *A Traffic of Dead Bodies: Anatomy and Embodied Social Identity in Nineteenth-Century America* (Princeton, N.J.: Princeton University Press, 2002), 83.

31 *They were often a rough-looking*: Stanley, *For Fear of Pain*, 166. Also described in "Horace Saltoun," *Cornhill Magazine* 3, no. 14 (Feb. 1861): 246.

31 *"wrought to such a degree"*: Advertisement, "Lancets," *Gazetteer and New Daily Advertiser*, Jan. 12, 1778, quoted in Alun Withey, *Technology, Self-Fashioning, and Politeness in Eighteenth-Century Britain: Refined Bodies* (London: Palgrave Pivot, 2015), 121.

32 *Older surgeons preferred the circular*: Stanley, *For Fear of Pain*, 81.

32 *Robert Liston—who was said*: Forbes Winslow, *Physic and Physicians: A Medical Sketch Book* (London: Longman, Orme, Brown, 1839), 2:362–63.

33 *"We do not think that the day"*: Quoted in Elisabeth Bennion, *Antique Medical Instruments* (Berkeley: University of California Press, 1979), 3.

34 *By 1788, there were 20,341 patients*: Erwin H. Ackerknecht, *Medicine at the Paris Hospital, 1794–1848* (Baltimore: Johns Hopkins Press, 1967), 15.

34 *Because they were often poor*: Ibid., 51.

34 *In the early decades of the nineteenth century*: Information sourced from Ann F. La Berge, "Debate as Scientific Practice in Nineteenth-Century Paris: The Controversy over the Microscope," *Perspectives on Science* 12, no. 4 (2004): 425–27.

35 *"spoke of the improvements introduced"*: A. E. Conrady, "The Unpublished Papers of J. J. Lister," *Journal of the Royal Microscopical Society* 29 (1913): 28–39. This letter is dated 1850, but I wonder if it is misdated, because the "Mr. Potter" he speaks of died in 1847.

35 *"By compressing a portion"*: Joseph Lister, "Observations on the Muscular Tissue of the Skin," *Quarterly Journal of Microscopical Science* 1 (1853): 264.

35 *Years later, Lister's supervisor*: Quoted in W. R. Merrington, *University*

College Hospital and Its Medical School: A History (London: Heinemann, 1976), 44.

2. HOUSES OF DEATH

37 *"What a charming task"*: D. Hayes Agnew, *Lecture Introductory to the One Hundred and Fifth Course of Instruction in the Medical Department of the University of Pennsylvania, Delivered Monday, October 10, 1870* (Philadelphia: R. P. King's Sons, 1870), 25, quoted in Sappol, *Traffic of Dead Bodies*, 75–76.

38 *Cadavers were left with their incised heads*: Dr. John Cheyne to Sir Edward Percival, Dec. 2, 1818, quoted in "Bodies for Dissection in Dublin," *British Medical Journal*, Jan. 16, 1943, 74, quoted in Richardson, *Death, Dissection, and the Destitute*, 97.

38 *"Not a sound could be heard"*: Quoted in Hale Bellot, *Notes on the History of University College, London with a Record of the Session 1886–7: Being the First Volume of the University College Gazette* (1887), 37.

38 *The cadaver tested the courage*: J. Marion Sims, *The Story of My Life* (New York: D. Appleton, 1884), 128–29, quoted in Sappol, *Traffic of Dead Bodies*, 78–79.

39 *"as though Death himself"*: Quoted in Peter Bloom, *The Life of Berlioz* (Cambridge, U.K.: Cambridge University Press, 1998), 14.

39 *Within the medical profession*: Robley Dunglison, *The Medical Student; or, Aids to the Study of Medicine . . .* (Philadelphia: Carey, Lea & Blanchard, 1837), 150.

40 *"forced the dead human body"*: W. W. Keen, *A Sketch of the Early History of Practical Anatomy: The Introductory Address to the Course of Lectures on Anatomy at the Philadelphia School of Anatomy . . .* (Philadelphia: J. B. Lippincott & Co., 1874), 3, quoted in Sappol, *Traffic of Bodies*, 77–78.

40 *It was a rite of passage*: Sappol, *Traffic of Dead Bodies*, 76.

40 *"Have you finished that leg yet?"*: Charles Dickens, *The Posthumous Papers of the Pickwick Club*, Chapter XXX (London: Chapman and Hall, 1868), 253.

40 *Today, we disparagingly call this*: William Hunter, Introductory Lecture to Students (ca. 1780), MS 55.182, St. Thomas' Hospital.

40 *The French anatomist Joseph-Guichard Duverney*: Patrick Mitchell, Lecture Notes Taken in Paris Mainly from the Lectures of Joseph

Guichard Duverney at the Jardin du Roi from 1697–8, MS 6.f.134, Wellcome Library, quoted in Lynda Payne, *With Words and Knives: Learning Medical Dispassion in Early Modern England* (Aldershot: Ashgate, 2007), 87.

40 Harper's New Monthly Magazine *condemned*: "Editor's Table," *Harper's New Monthly Magazine*, April 1854, 692.

41 *"Not a single session has passed"*: W. T. Gairdner, *Introductory Address at the Public Opening of the Medical Session 1866–67 in the University of Glasgow* (Glasgow: Maclehose, 1866), 22, quoted in M. Anne Crowther and Marguerite W. Dupree, *Medical Lives in the Age of Surgical Revolution* (Cambridge, U.K.: Cambridge University Press, 2007), 45.

41 *Mortality rates among medical students*: Robert Woods, "Physician, Heal Thyself: The Health and Mortality of Victorian Doctors," *Social History of Medicine* 9 (1996): 1–30.

41 *Between 1843 and 1859*: "Medical Education," *New York Medical Inquirer* 1 (1830): 130, cited in Sappol, *Traffic of Dead Bodies*, 80.

41 *"God help you all"*: Thomas Pettigrew, *Biographical Memoirs of the Most Celebrated Physicians, Surgeons, etc., etc., Who Have Contributed to the Advancement of Medical Science* (London: Fisher, Son, 1839–40), 2:4–5, quoted in Stanley, *For Fear of Pain*, 159. A contemporary claimed that Abernethy added, "What is to become of you?" Winslow, *Physic and Physicians*, 1:119.

42 *"hideous traces of its power"*: Thomas Babington Macaulay, *The History of England from the Accession of James II* (London: Longman, Green, Longman, Roberts, & Green, 1864), 73.

42 *His friend and fellow lodger John Hodgkin*: See Fisher, *Joseph Lister*, 40–41.

43 *"I will be with thee"*: Hodgkin, Remembrance of Lister's Youth.

43 *"cloud of seriousness"*: John Rudd Leeson, *Lister as I Knew Him* (New York: William Wood, 1927), 58–60.

43 *Throughout Victoria's reign*: Janet Oppenheim, *Shattered Nerves: Doctors, Patients, and Depression in Victorian England* (Oxford: Oxford University Press, 1991), 110–11.

44 *"The things that sometimes distress"*: Quoted in Fisher, *Joseph Lister*, 42. Letter from Joseph Jackson Lister to Joseph Lister, July 1, 1848, MS 6965/7, Wellcome Library.

45 *These included a bladder*: Cashbook, Dec. 1, 1849, MS 6981, Wellcome Library.

45 *After the first year of medical school*: Quoted in Fisher, *Joseph Lister*, 47. Although there is no direct mention of his mental state during this period, it's possible that he passed up this opportunity on the advice of his father, who told him to tackle his studies in moderation in light of his breakdown two years earlier.

45 *The best that can be said*: Adrian Teal, *The Gin Lane Gazette* (London: Unbound, 2014).

46 *Some only admitted patients*: Elisabeth Bennion, *Antique Medical Instruments* (Berkeley: University of California Press, 1979), 13.

46 *"a soldier has more chance of survival"*: James Y. Simpson, "Our Existing System of Hospitalism and Its Effects," *Edinburgh Medical Journal*, March 1869, 818.

46 *In spite of token efforts*: Youngson, *Scientific Revolution*, 23–24.

46 *In 1825, visitors to St. George's Hospital*: F. B. Smith, *The People's Health, 1830–1910* (London: Croom Helm, 1979), 262, cited in Stanley, *For Fear of Pain*, 139.

46 *The smell was so offensive*: Youngson, *Scientific Revolution*, 24.

47 *In England and Wales in the 1840s*: Statistic quoted ibid., 40.

48 *His most successful book*: Ibid., 65.

48 *"It is long since"*: John Eric Erichsen, *On the Study of Surgery: An Address Introductory to the Course of Surgery, Delivered at University College, London, at the Opening of Session 1850–1851* (London: Taylor, Walton & Maberly, 1850), 8.

49 *"like a head and trunk"*: Quoted in Jacob Smith, *The Thrill Makers: Celebrity, Masculinity, and Stunt Performance* (Berkeley: University of California Press, 2012), 53.

49 *Unbeknownst to Barnum*: Although Barnum's first "What Is It?" exhibit was a failure, his follow-up attempt in 1860 was a wild success in the United States. It came on the heels of Charles Darwin's *Origin of Species*, which put the question of the "missing link" into everyone's mind. Barnum's second "What Is It?" was an African American man named William Henry Johnson. As the historian Stephen Asma points out, one wonders if the racist dimension of the exhibit played better to an American audience on the cusp of a civil war than it did

in England, where slavery had been abolished decades earlier. Stephen T. Asma, *On Monsters: An Unnatural History of Our Worst Fears* (Oxford: Oxford University Press, 2009), 138.

49 *Despite this initial bungle*: "John Phillips Potter FRCS," *The Lancet*, May 29, 1847, 576.

49 *"be presented to Dr. Liston"*: "Obituary Notices," *South Australian Register*, July 28, 1847, 2.

49 *"bequeathed his body"*: "Death from Dissecting," *Daily News* (London), May 25, 1847, 3.

49 *Potter, who had proven himself*: "John Phillips Potter FRCS," 576–77.

50 *"It seems as though the thigh-bones"*: *Courier*, Oct. 13, 1847, 4. See also "Dissection of the Man Monkey," *Stirling Observer*, April 29, 1847, 3.

50 *"a most melancholy and disheartening instance"*: "John Phillips Potter FRCS," 576.

51 *His death was felt deeply*: Merrington, *University College Hospital*, 65.

51 *By the end of the 1840s*: Ibid., 49.

52 *For the first time in his life*: Godlee, *Lord Lister*, 20.

52 *He also led a scathing attack*: Quoted in Fisher, *Joseph Lister*, 50–51, 307.

52 *His mother, Isabella, had suffered*: Joseph Jackson Lister to Joseph Lister, Oct. 9, 1838, MS 6965/1, Wellcome Library.

53 *"unreasoned dread of wet feet"*: Leeson, *Lister as I Knew Him*, 48–49.

53 *"progress in the public practice"*: James Y. Simpson, *Hospitalism: Its Effects on the Results of Surgical Operations, etc. Part I* (Edinburgh: Oliver and Boyd, 1869), 4.

54 *"the poison of atmospheric impurity"*: Royal Commission for Enquiring into the State of Large Towns and Populous Districts, *Parliamentary Papers* (1844), 17, quoted in Stephen Halliday, "Death and Miasma in Victorian London: An Obstinate Belief," *British Medical Journal*, Dec. 22, 2001, 1469–71.

54 *While many medical practitioners*: See Michael Worboys, *Spreading Germs: Disease Theories and Medical Practice in Britain, 1865–1900* (Cambridge, U.K.: Cambridge University Press, 2000), 28.

55 *"at any season of the year"*: John Eric Erichsen, *On Hospitalism and the Causes of Death After Operations* (London: Longmans, Green, 1874), 36.

55 *While comparing mortality rates*: James Y. Simpson, *Hospitalism: Its Effects on the Results of Surgical Operations, etc. Part II* (Edinburgh: Oliver and Boyd, 1869), 20–24.

55 *University College Hospital had a swift*: UCH/MR/1/63, University College London Archives.

3. THE SUTURED GUT

57 *"We should ask ourselves"*: Quoted in Bransby Blake Cooper, *The Life of Sir Astley Cooper* (London: J. W. Parker, 1843), 2:207.

57 *Other wards had recently installed gaslit*: R. S. Pilcher, "Lister's Medical School," *British Journal of Surgery* 54 (1967): 422. See also blueprints of building found in Merrington, *University College Hospital*, 78–79.

57 *One of Erichsen's patients*: Pilcher, "Lister's Medical School," 422.

58 *He set the candle down*: I am hugely indebted to Ruth Richardson and Bryan Rhodes for the information in this chapter. They were the first to discover this obscure surgery that Lister had performed at the very beginning of his career. See Ruth Richardson and Bryan Rhodes, "Joseph Lister's First Operation," *Notes and Records of the Royal Society of London* 67, no. 4 (2013): 375–85.

58 *"does agree to part with my wife"*: C. Kenny, "Wife-Selling in England," *Law Quarterly Review* 45 (1929): 496.

58 *In another instance, a journalist*: "Letters Patent Have Passed the Great Seal of Ireland . . . ," *Times*, July 18, 1797, 3.

59 *Between 1800 and 1850*: Lawrence Stone, *Road to Divorce: England, 1530–1987* (Oxford: Oxford University Press, 1992), 429.

59 *The editor of* The Times *criticized*: "The Disproportion Between the Punishments," *Times*, Aug. 24, 1846, 4.

59 *"It is evident to all"*: Harriet Taylor Mill and John Stuart Mill [unheaded leader—Assault Law], *Morning Chronicle*, May 31, 1850, 4.

59 *This was the world in which Julia*: The account of what happened to Julia Sullivan (unless stated otherwise) comes from Proceedings of the Central Criminal Court, Sept. 15, 1851, 27–32, available online at https://www.oldbaileyonline.org.

61 *The drunken perpetrator ranted*: "Central Criminal Court, Sept. 17," *Times*, Sept. 18, 1851, 7.

62 *In general, a sick person*: Stanley, *For Fear of Pain*, 136.

62 *In 1845, King's College Hospital*: Ibid.

62 *In 1835,* The Times *reported*: T.W.H., "To the Editor of the Times," *Times*, July 11, 1835, 3.

62 *Julia Sullivan was lucky*: Details of this operation are largely derived from Lister's testimony in the Old Bailey records and John Eric Erichsen, "University College Hospital: Wound of the Abdomen; Protrusion and Perforation of the Intestines and Mesentery; Recovery," *The Lancet*, Nov. 1, 1851, 414–15.

64 *Very early in Lister's residency*: "Mirror on the Practice of Medicine and Surgery in the Hospitals of London: University College Hospital," *The Lancet*, Jan. 11, 1851, 41–42.

65 *The surgeon Benjamin Travers*: Benjamin Travers, "A Case of Wound with Protrusion of the Stomach," *Edinburgh Journal of Medical Science* 1 (1826): 81–84.

66 *Later in 1851, her case*: Erichsen, "University College Hospital: Wound of the Abdomen; Protrusion and Perforation of the Intestines and Mesentery; Recovery," 415. Two years later, Erichsen published a textbook, *The Science and Art of Surgery*, in which he refers to the stabbing. He fails to credit Lister's heroic surgical efforts, without which Julia Sullivan would most certainly have died that nerve-racking evening. Unfortunately, the casebooks relating to Erichsen's female patients have since been lost, so we don't have Lister's own notes on Julia Sullivan's operation.

67 *"Nothing is so likely to strike"*: Charles Dickens, *Sketches by Boz: Illustrative of Every-Day Life and Every-Day People, with Forty Illustrations* (London: Chapman & Hall, 1839), 210.

4. THE ALTAR OF SCIENCE

71 *"Men may rise on stepping-stones"*: Alfred, Lord Tennyson, *In Memoriam A.H.H.* (London: Edward Moxon, 1850) I, lines 3–4.

72 *There were some incredibly lucky cases*: John Eric Erichsen, *The Science and Art of Surgery: Being a Treatise on Surgical Injuries, Diseases, and Preparations* (London: Walton and Maberly, 1853), 698–99.

72 *Between 1834 and 1850*: Stanley, *For Fear of Pain*, 73.

73 *"broken glass or porcelain"*: [The Annual Report of the Committee of the Charing Cross Hospital], *Spectator* 10 (London, 1837), 58.

73 *These accidents often involved children*: Accident Report for Martha Appleton, A Scavenger, Aug. 1859, HO 45/6753, National Archives.

73 *There was a fifty-six-year-old painter*: Notes of cases taken by Lister, student number 351, for the Fellowe's Clinical Medal at University College Hospital 1851, MS0021/4/4 (3), Royal College of Surgeons of England.

73 *"Dust does not kill suddenly"*: Quoted in Jack London, *People of the Abyss* (New York: Macmillan 1903), 258. See also John Thomas Arlidge, *The Hygiene, Diseases, and Mortality of Occupations* (London: Percival, 1892).

74 *Over the summer, two people*: For more on treatment of scurvy in the eighteenth and nineteenth centuries, see Mark Harrison, "Scurvy on Sea and Land: Political Economy and Natural History, c. 1780–c. 1850," *Journal for Maritime Research (Print)* 15, no. 1 (2013): 7–15. It wasn't until 1928 that the biochemist Albert Szent-Györgyi isolated from adrenal glands the substance that enables the body to use carbohydrates, fats, and protein efficiently. It would be another four years before Charles Glen King discovered vitamin C in his laboratory and concluded that it was identical to the substance that Szent-Györgyi described—providing clear links between scurvy and vitamin C deficiencies.

74 *"an eccentric gentleman"*: "Origin of the No Nose Club," *Star*, Feb. 18, 1874, 3.

75 *At University College Hospital*: Notes of cases taken by Lister, student number 351, for the Fellowe's Clinical Medal at University College Hospital, 1851, MS0021/4/4 (3), Royal College of Surgeons of England.

75 *Another case involved a twenty-one-year-old*: Ibid.

77 *An artificial leech*: Robert Ellis, *Official Descriptive and Illustrated Catalogue of the Great Exhibition of the Works of Industry of All Nations, 1851* (London: W. Clowes and Sons, 1851), 3:1070.

77 *One exhibitor from Paris*: Ibid., 1170.

77 *"It is a wonderful place"*: Margaret Smith, ed., *The Letters of Charlotte Brontë, with a Selection of Letters by Family and Friends* (Oxford: Clarendon Press, 2000), 2:630.

78 *"I even saw . . . a valve"*: Quoted in Godlee, *Lord Lister*, 28.

78 *After he had caught a lamprey*: Drawings of Lamprey, March 31, April 2,

April 7, 1852, MS0021/4/4 (2/6), Royal College of Surgeons of England.

79 *"This instrument seems to have been"*: Quoted in Fisher, *Joseph Lister*, 48.

79 *"As a student at University College"*: Joseph Lister, "The Huxley Lecture on Early Researches Leading Up to the Antiseptic System of Surgery," *The Lancet,* Oct. 6, 1900, 985.

80 *It would take another hundred years*: Jackie Rosenhek, "The Art of Artificial Insemination," *Doctor's Review*, Oct. 2013, accessed May 14, 2015, http://www.doctorsreview.com/history/history-artificial-insemination/.

81 *In 1852, Lister made his first*: A. E. Best, "Reflections on Joseph Lister's Edinburgh Experiments on Vaso-motor Control," *Medical History* 14, no. 1 (1970): 10–30. See also Edward R. Howard, "Joseph Lister: His Contributions to Early Experimental Physiology," *Notes and Records of the Royal Society of London* 67, no. 3 (2013): 191–98.

81 *Lister carefully teased portions of tissue*: Joseph Lister, "Observations on the Contractile Tissue of the Iris," *Quarterly Journal of Microscopical Science* 1 (1853): 8–11.

82 *"the wound swells, the skin retracts"*: John Bell, *The Principles of Surgery*, 2nd ed., abridged by J. Augustine Smith (New York: Collins, 1812), 26–27.

82 *The first English descriptions*: Reported in T. Trotter, *Medicina Nautica* (London: Longman, Hurst, Rees, and Orme, 1797–1803), cited in I. Loudon, "Necrotising Fasciitis, Hospital Gangrene, and Phagedena," *The Lancet*, Nov. 19, 1994, 1416.

83 *"whole length of the urethra"*: Quoted in Loudon, "Necrotising Fasciitis," 1416.

83 *"Without the circle of infected walls"*: Bell, *Principles of Surgery*, 28.

83 *"This hospital gangrene"*: James Syme, *The Principles of Surgery* (Edinburgh: MacLaughlan & Stewart, 1832), 69.

83 *When outbreaks occurred*: Worboys, *Spreading Germs*, 75.

84 *"As a rule . . . a perfectly healthy"*: Joseph Lister, "The Huxley Lecture by Lord Lister, F.R.C.S., President of the Royal Society," *British Medical Journal*, Oct. 6, 1900, 969.

84 *Only in one case*: Ibid.

85 *"I examined microscopically"*: Ibid.

85   *"the allurements of medicine"*: Godlee, *Lord Lister*, 28.

85   *"Had it not been for you"*: Ibid., 21.

86   *"I think it as well"*: Ibid., 22.

86   *"I care but little comparatively for this"*: Lister to Godlee, reply to a letter dated Nov. 28, 1852, MS 6970/1, Wellcome Library.

86   *It was true that Lister*: Notes of cases taken by Lister, student no. 351, for the Fellowe's Clinical Medal at University College Hospital 1851, MS0021/4/4 (3), Royal College of Surgeons of England.

5. THE NAPOLEON OF SURGERY

89   *"Were I to place a man"*: William Hunter, *Two Introductory Lectures, Delivered by Dr. William Hunter, to his Last Course of Anatomical Lectures, at his Theatre in Windmill-Street* (London: Printed by order of the trustees, for J. Johnson, 1784), 73.

90   *"never unnecessarily wasted a word"*: Quoted in Alexander Peddie, "Dr. John Brown: His Life and Work; with Narrative Sketches of James Syme in the Old Minto House Hospital and Dispensary Days; Being the Harveian Society Oration, Delivered 11th April 1890," *Edinburgh Medical Journal* 35, pt. 2 (Jan.–June 1890): 1058.

91   *"Had it not been for"*: Alexander Miles, *The Edinburgh School of Surgery Before Lister* (London: A. & C. Black, 1918), 181–82.

93   *Over a third of these households*: A. J. K. Cairncross, ed., *Census of Scotland, 1861–1931* (Cambridge, U.K., 1954).

93   *Within these quarters, crime rates soared*: "Statistics of Crime in Edinburgh," *Caledonian Mercury* (Edinburgh), Jan. 21, 1856.

94   *"foully tainted, and rendered almost unendurable"*: James Begg, *Happy Homes for Working Men, and How to Get Them* (London: Cassell, Petter & Galpin, 1866), 159.

95   *In one instance, a father grieving*: Ibid.

96   *"I shall not have, as in London"*: Quoted in Godlee, *Lord Lister*, 31.

96   *"There, gentlemen, is what"*: Quoted in John D. Comrie, *History of Scottish Medicine*, 2nd ed., vol. 2 (London: Published for the Wellcome Historical Medical Museum by Baillière, Tindall & Cox, 1932), 596.

97   *"Huh, so you've come"*: Ibid., 596–97.

97   *In that same year*: The site of the hospital is now occupied by the Royal Museum of Scotland.

98 *"Don't support quackery and humbug"*: Quoted in R. G. Williams Jr., "James Syme of Edinburgh," *Historical Bulletin: Notes and Abstracts Dealing with Medical History* 16, no. 2 (1951): 27.

98 *"tell me that you wish"*: Ibid., 28.

98 *Indeed, at times, Edinburgh*: For more on the duel, see Stanley, *For Fear of Pain*, 37.

99 *It was massive*: Bill Yule, *Matrons, Medics, and Maladies* (East Linton: Tuckwell Press, 1999), 3–5.

100 *"If the day were twice"*: Quoted in Godlee, *Lord Lister*, 30.

100 *"My present opportunities are teaching"*: Ibid., 34.

100 *A few days later, Syme*: Fisher makes this point in his book *Joseph Lister*, 60–61.

101 *"If the love of surgery is a proof"*: Godlee, *Lord Lister*, 35.

101 "Nullius jurare in verba magistri": Ibid., 37.

101 *"I am pleased to be"*: Ibid., 37, 38.

101 *"Why! You must be"*: Letter from George Buchanan to Joseph Lister, Dec. 10–11, 1853, MS 6970/3, Wellcome Library.

102 *"Two lives . . . depended upon the slow"*: G. T. Wrench, *Lord Lister: His Life and Work* (London: Unwin, 1913), 45.

102 *"there was written the anxiety"*: Ibid., 46.

103 *"Even now I cannot, without a shudder"*: James Syme, *Observations in Clinical Surgery* (Edinburgh: Edmonston and Douglas, 1861), 160.

103 *The seconds ticked by*: Wrench, *Lord Lister*, 47.

104 *Lister quickly gained the respect*: Hector Charles Cameron, *Joseph Lister: The Friend of Man* (London: William Heinemann Medical Books, 1948), 34.

105 *"drunken night nurses"*: Nightingale to R. G. Whitfield, Nov. 8, 1856 (LMA) H1/ST/NC1/58/6, London Metropolitan Archives, quoted in Lynn McDonald, ed., *Florence Nightingale: Extending Nursing* (Waterloo, Ont.: Wilfrid Laurier University Press, 2009), 303.

105 *The poet W. E. Henley*: Poem quoted in Cameron, *Joseph Lister*, 34–35.

105 *"[In] high dudgeon, she snatched"*: Ibid., 35.

106 *The Cat's Nick cut*: John Beddoe, *Memories of Eighty Years* (Bristol: J. W. Arrowsmith, 1910), 56.

106 *"I feel giddy"*: Ibid.

106 *"whirled down the talus"*: Ibid.

107 *"Eh, Doketur Bedie!"*: Ibid., 56–57.

107 *"If I had killed my friend"*: Ibid., 55.

6. THE FROG'S LEGS

109 *"Everywhere questions arose"*: Quoted in William J. Sinclair, *Semmel-weis: His Life and His Doctrine: A Chapter in the History of Medicine* (Manchester: University Press, 1909), 46.

110 *"We had, as you know"*: "The Late Richard Mackenzie MD," *Association Medical Journal* (1854): 1023, 1024.

111 *"Many were struck down"*: Ibid., 1024. For more on Mackenzie, see also *Medical Times & Gazette* 2 (1854): 446–47.

111 *During the two-and-a-half-year conflict*: Matthew Smallman-Raynora and Andrew D. Cliff, "The Geographical Spread of Cholera in the Crimean War: Epidemic Transmission in the Camp Systems of the British Army of the East, 1854–55," *Journal of Historical Geography* 30 (2004): 33. See also Army Medical Department, *The Medical and Surgical History of the British Army Which Served in Turkey and the Crimea During the War Against Russia in the Years 1854–55–56*, vol. 1 (London: HMSO, 1858).

112 *"the only passport"*: Quoted in Frieda Marsden Sandwith, *Surgeon Compassionate: The Story of Dr. William Marsden, Founder of the Royal Free and Royal Marsden Hospitals* (London: P. Davies, 1960), 70.

113 *"The new Surgeon will be thrown"*: Letter from William Sharpey to James Syme, Dec. 1, 1854, MS 6979/21, Wellcome Library.

114 *"Thou art now at liberty"*: Letter from Joseph Jackson Lister to Joseph Lister, Dec. 5, 1854, MS 6965/11, Wellcome Library.

114 *"If a man is not to take"*: Ibid., 40.

115 *"premises that are in their character"*: Joseph Jackson Lister to Joseph Lister, April 16, 1855, MS 6965/13, Wellcome Library.

115 *In September, he collected his first fee*: Godlee, *Lord Lister*, 43.

115 *As well-appointed as Lister's*: Description of Millbank House can be found in Robert Paterson, *Memorials of the Life of James Syme, Professor of Clinical Surgery in the University of Edinburgh, etc.* (Edinburgh: Edmonston & Douglas, 1874), 293–95. See also Wrench, *Lord Lister*, 42–44.

116 *In a letter back home*: Joseph Lister to Rickman Godlee, Aug. 4, 1855, MS 6969/4, Wellcome Library.

117 *"Thy dear mother tells me"*: Joseph Jackson Lister to Joseph Lister, March 25, 1853, MS6965/8, Wellcome Library.

117 *"As Syme was a stalking"*: Quoted in Fisher, *Joseph Lister*, 63. Poem, "'Tis of a winemerchant who in London did dwell," by John Beddoe, David Christison, and Patrick Heron Watson, May 15, 1854, MS6979/9, Wellcome Library.

118 *"I would not allow"*: Letter from Joseph Jackson Lister to Joseph Lister, July 24, 1855, MS6965/14, Wellcome Library.

118 *"attend the worship of 'Friends'"*: Joseph Jackson Lister to Joseph Lister, Oct. 18, 1855, MS6965/16, Wellcome Library.

119 *"My preference like thine"*: Joseph Jackson Lister to Joseph Lister, Feb. 23, 1856, MS6965/20, Wellcome Library.

119 *The wedding gifts began*: Ibid.

119 *With Agnes's considerable dowry*: Joseph Jackson and James Syme negotiated a settlement for the marriage. Syme gave two thousand pounds in securities and two thousand pounds in cash, and Lister's father also contributed to the union. For more information, see Fisher, *Joseph Lister*, 80.

119 *well provided with a sink*: Ibid., letter from Joseph Lister to Isabella Lister, Jan. ?–6, 1856, MS6968/2, Wellcome Library.

119 *"out of consideration"*: Quoted in Fisher, *Joseph Lister*, 81.

119 *"Lister is one who, I believe"*: Quoted in Sir Hector Clare Cameron, *Lord Lister 1827–1912: An Oration* (Glasgow: J. Maclehose, 1914), 9. Some sources contest whether this was delivered at Lister's wedding reception or at a later date.

120 *In the 1850s, however*: Youngson, *Scientific Revolution*, 34–35.

120 *Moreover, there was a debate*: Worboys, *Spreading Germs*, 76.

120 *"felt that the early stages"*: Quoted in Godlee, *Lord Lister*, 43.

121 *"the patient is kept"*: Robert Liston, *Practical Surgery*, 3rd ed. (London: John Churchill, 1840), 31.

123 *"The bandages and instruments"*: *Year-Book of Medicine, Surgery, and Their Allied Sciences for 1862* (London: Printed for the New Sydenham Society, 1863), 213, quoted in Youngson, *Scientific Revolution*, 38.

123 *During the first year*: Fisher, *Joseph Lister*, 84.

124 *Until this time, Lister*: Later in life, Lister said that he considered his research into the nature of inflammation to be an "essential preliminary" to his conception of the antiseptic principle and insisted these early findings be included in any memorial volume of his work. In 1905, when he was seventy-eight years old, he wrote, "If my works are read when I am gone, these will be the ones most highly thought of" (quoted ibid., 89).

124 *Lister's investigations into inflammation*: Edward R. Howard, "Joseph Lister: His Contributions to Early Experimental Physiology," *Notes and Records of the Royal Society of London* 67, no. 3 (2013): 191–98.

125 *"the arteries, which had previously"*: Quoted in Fisher, *Joseph Lister*, 87. Joseph Lister, "An Inquiry Regarding the Parts of the Nervous System Which Regulate the Contractions of the Arteries," *Philosophical Transactions of the Royal Society of London* 148 (1858): 612–13.

125 *"The blood had ceased to move"*: Ibid., 614.

126 *"one third had to be spoken"*: Quoted in Godlee, *Lord Lister*, 61.

126 *"a certain amount of inflammation"*: Joseph Lister, "On the Early Stages of Inflammation," *Philosophical Transactions of the Royal Society of London* 148 (1858): 700.

126 *In opposition to Wharton Jones*: Howard, "Joseph Lister," 194.

126 *These early studies were crucial*: Ibid.

126 *"I am ready to ask"*: Joseph Jackson Lister to Joseph Lister, Jan. 31, 1857, MS6965/26, Wellcome Library.

7. CLEANLINESS AND COLD WATER

129 *"The surgeon is like the husbandman"*: Richard Volkmann, "Die moderne Chirurgie," *Sammlung klinischer Vortrage*, quoted in Sir Rickman John Godlee, *Lord Lister*, 2nd ed. (London: Macmillan and Co., 1918), 123.

130 *"Dr. Lawrie . . . is in such a state"*: Quoted in Godlee, *Lord Lister*, 77.

130 *Moreover, Lister assumed*: Ibid., 78.

130 *"I should very much regret"*: Ibid., 78, 77.

131 *"strict regard for accuracy"*: Ibid., 82.

131 *Then, in December, Lister received*: This letter is alluded to in Godlee, *Lord Lister*, 80. I couldn't discover the writer of the letter, and subsequent authors such as Fisher make no mention of it.

131 *"inform us which candidate"*: *Glasgow Herald*, Jan. 18, 1860, 3.

131 *The protest grew, with William Sharpey*: Fisher, *Joseph Lister*, 97.

131 *"At last the welcome news"*: Quoted in Godlee, *Lord Lister*, 81.

132 *The Glaswegian medical community*: Cameron, *Joseph Lister*, 46.

132 *"We ought to be men and gentlemen"*: Quoted in Christopher Lawrence, "Incommunicable Knowledge: Science, Technology, and the Clinical Art in Britain, 1850–1914," *Journal of Contemporary History* 20, no. 4 (1985): 508.

132 *Now, as he stood before the audience*: Letter quoted in Godlee, *Lord Lister*, 88–89.

132 *But as he began to speak*: Based on an account told by Cameron, *Joseph Lister*, 47–49.

133 *When Lister joined the faculty*: Fisher, *Joseph Lister*, 98; Crowther and Dupree, *Medical Lives in the Age of Surgical Revolution*, 61–62.

133 *Of these, over half*: Godlee, *Lord Lister*, 92.

133 *While Edinburgh had allocated*: Crowther and Dupree, *Medical Lives in the Age of Surgical Revolution*, 63.

133 *He decided to invest*: The renovations are discussed by Godlee, *Lord Lister*, 90.

133 *"How nice it looks"*: Ibid., 91.

133 *The refurbishments had an instantaneous effect*: Ibid.

134 *He opened with a quotation*: Ibid.

134 *Again, he had the room*: Ibid.

134 *"I now feel"*: Ibid., 93.

134 *"The game may be"*: Ibid., 92.

136 *"Stop, stop, Mr. Lister"*: Sir Hector Clare Cameron, *Reminiscences of Lister and of His Work in the Wards of the Glasgow Royal Infirmary, 1860–1869* (Glasgow: Jackson, Wylie & Co., 1927), 9.

136 *"I have seen human degradation"*: J. C. Symons, quoted in Friedrich Engels, *The Condition of the Working Class in England*, trans. and ed. W. O. Henderson and W. H. Chaloner, 2nd ed. (Oxford: Blackwell, 1971), 45.

137 *William Duff*: "Accident," *Fife Herald*, Jan. 12, 1865, 3.

137 *Joseph Neille*: "Uphall—Gunpowder Accident," *Scotsman*, April 3, 1865, 2.

138 *"Permit us to express"*: Quoted in Godlee, *Lord Lister*, 92.

138 *In fact, it was nearly two years*: Quoted in John D. Comrie, *History of Scottish Medicine*, 2nd ed., vol. 2 (London: Published for the Wellcome Historical Medical Museum by Baillière, Tindall & Cox, 1932), 459.

138 *Originally, the hospital contained*: Fisher, *Joseph Lister*, 107.

139 *Despite having been built months earlier*: Cameron, *Reminiscences of Lister*, 11.

139 *"Its newness had not saved it"*: Cameron, *Joseph Lister*, 52.

139 *"uppermost tier of a multitude"*: Godlee, *Lord Lister*, 130, 129.

139 *"When almost every wound"*: Ibid., 55.

139 *He refused to use*: Leeson, *Lister as I Knew Him*, 51, 103.

140 *He also recommended*: Ibid., 87.

140 *"How can you have such cruel disregard"*: Ibid., 111.

140 *"Every patient, even the most degraded"*: Ibid., 53.

140 *Lister's house surgeon Douglas Guthrie*: Douglas Guthrie, *Lord Lister: His Life and Doctrine* (Edinburgh: E. & S. Livingstone, 1949), 63–64.

141 *One of Lister's house surgeons*: Leeson, *Lister as I Knew Him*, 19.

142 *"Shall we charge for the blood"*: Quoted in Fisher, *Joseph Lister*, 111.

142 *"the influence exerted upon it"*: Joseph Lister, "The Croonian Lecture: On the Coagulation of the Blood," *Proceedings of the Royal Society of London* 12 (1862–63): 609.

142 *Lister designed and patented*: Guthrie, *Lord Lister*, 45–46.

142 *In August 1863, Lister performed surgery*: Joseph Lister, "On the Excision of the Wrist for Caries," *The Lancet*, March 25, 1865, 308–12.

143 *"11 P.M. Query"*: Quoted in Fisher, *Joseph Lister*, 122.

144 *"Lister always looked upon himself"*: Godlee, *Lord Lister*, 110.

144 *"The thought that thou wilt"*: Joseph Jackson Lister to Joseph Lister, Nov. 30, 1864, MS6965/40, Wellcome Library.

144 *Lister pledged to write*: Godlee, *Lord Lister*, 111.

144 *"As thee say, I have now arrived"*: Quoted ibid., 105.

145 *Between 1795 and 1860*: Youngson, *Scientific Revolution*, 130.

145 *Over the course of three years*: Peter M. Dunn, "Dr. Alexander Gordon (1752–99) and Contagious Puerperal Fever," *Archives of Disease in Childhood: Fetal and Neonatal Edition* 78, no. 3 (1998): F232.

145–46 *In his report published in 1795*: Alexander Gordon, *A Treatise on the Epidemic Puerperal Fever of Aberde*en (London: Printed for G. G. and J. Robinson, 1795), 3, 63, 99.

146 *The second person to make*: Youngson, *Scientific Revolution*, 132.

146 *And then there was Ignaz Semmelweis*: Ibid.

147 *In April 1847, the rate was 18.3 percent*: Ignaz Semmelweis, *Etiology, Concept, and Prophylaxis of Childbed Fever* (1861), trans. K. Kodell Carter (Madison: University of Wisconsin Press, 1983), 131.

148 *In fact, Semmelweis's methods and theories*: Youngson, *Scientific Revolution*, 134.

148 *"Semmelweis's name was never mentioned"*: Quoted in Cameron, *Joseph Lister*, 57.

148 *In one week, Lister lost*: Cameron, *Reminiscences of Lister*, 11.

148 *His house surgeon said*: Cameron, *Joseph Lister*, 54.

148 *"It is a common observation"*: Ibid., 54–55.

148 *Then, at the end of 1864*: Some accounts list the year as 1865, others as 1864. I've taken this date from Sir William Watson Cheyne, *Lister and His Achievement* (London: Longmans, Green, 1925), 8.

8. THEY'RE ALL DEAD

151 *"No Scientific subject can be so important"*: George Henry Lewes, *The Physiology of Common Life*, vol. 2 (Edinburgh: W. Blackwood, 1859–60), 452.

151 *Upon inquiring after the welfare*: "Letters, News, etc.," *The Lancet*, April 26, 1834, 176, quoted in Stanley, *For Fear of Pain*, 152. This story is from earlier in the nineteenth century but holds true for the 1860s. Italics mine.

152 *There had already been three*: Margaret Pelling, *Cholera, Fever, and English Medicine, 1825–1865* (Oxford: Oxford University Press, 1978), 2.

152 *Although non-contagionists could point*: Gaw, *"Time to Heal,"* 19.

152 *"a living organism of a distinct species"*: Quoted in R. J. Morris, *Cholera, 1832: The Social Response to an Epidemic* (New York: Holmes & Meier, 1976), 207.

152 *"the poisons of specific contagious diseases"*: William Budd, "Investigations of Epidemic and Epizootic Diseases," *British Medical Journal*, Sept. 24, 1864, 356, quoted in Gaw, *"Time to Heal,"* 24. Interestingly, Budd thought that the cholera poison could be carried in the air but believed

it spread not by inhalation but by the ingestion of aerially contaminated food and water.

152 *"All discharges from the sick"*: W. Budd, "Cholera: Its Cause and Prevention," *British Medical Journal*, March 2, 1855, 207.

153 *"The feculence rolled up in clouds"*: M. Faraday, "The State of the Thames, Letter to the Editor," *Times*, July 9, 1855, 8.

154 *"bent upon investigating the matter"*: *Times*, June 18, 1858, 9.

155 *"complex milieu composed of two isomers"*: Quoted in Patrice Debré, *Louis Pasteur*, trans. Elborg Forster (Baltimore: Johns Hopkins University Press, 1998), 96.

156 *Pasteur began making daily visits*: Ibid., 87.

156 *If it was corrupted, the yeast*: René Dubos, *Pasteur and Modern Science*, ed. Thomas D. Brock (Washington, D.C.: ASM Press, 1998), 32.

157–58 *"Never will the doctrine of spontaneous generation"*: René Vallery-Radot, *The Life of Pasteur*, trans. Mrs. R. L. Devonshire (Westminster: Archibald Constable & Co, 1902), 1:142, in Godlee, *Lord Lister*, 176.

158 *"the world of the infinitely small"*: Quoted in Sherwin B. Nuland, *Doctors: The Biography of Medicine* (New York: Vintage Books, 1989), 363.

158 *"I am afraid that the experiments"*: Quoted in Vallery-Radot, *The Life of Pasteur*, vol. I, 129.

158 *"The applications of my ideas"*: Debré, *Louis Pasteur*, 260.

158 *"Life directs the work of death"*: Ibid., 110.

158 *"How I wish I had"*: Ibid., 260.

159 *"[By] applying the knowledge"*: Thomas Spencer Wells, "Some Causes of Excessive Mortality After Surgical Operations," *British Medical Journal*, Oct. 1, 1864, 386.

159 *Unfortunately, Wells failed to make the impact*: Fisher, *Joseph Lister*, 134.

160 *"When I read Pasteur's article"*: "Meeting of the International Medical Congress," *The Boston Medical and Surgical Journal* 95 (Sept. 14, 1876): 328.

160 *"It was a great part of the care"*: *The Lancet*, Aug. 24, 1867, 234.

160 *Unfortunately, while blood poisoning*: See Fisher, *Joseph Lister*, 131.

161 *"held the limb in one hand"*: Quoted ibid., 130.

161 *Frederick Crace Calvert*: John. K. Crellin, "The Disinfectant Studies by F. Crace Calvert and the Introduction of Phenol as a Germicide," *Vorträge der Hauptversammlung der internationalen Gesellschaft für Geschichte*

der Pharmazie; International Society for the History of Pharmacy, Meeting, 1965, London 28 (1966): 3.

161 *"struck with an account"*: Joseph Lister, "On a New Method of Treating Compound Fracture, Abscess, etc., with Observations on the Conditions of Suppuration," *The Lancet*, March 16, 1867, 327.

162 *It was first discovered in 1834*: Fisher, *Joseph Lister*, 134.

162 *"It proved unsuccessful, in consequence"*: Lister, "On a New Method of Treating Compound Fracture," 328.

162 *And because simple fractures did not*: Joseph Lister, "On the Principles of Antiseptic Surgery," in *Internationale Beiträge zur wissenschaftlichen Medizin: Festschrift, Rudolf Virchow gewidmet zur Vollendung seines 70. Lebensjahres* (Berlin: August Hirschwald, 1891), 3:262.

163 *This particular kind of break*: Although Kelly had been suffering from a similar type of fracture, Lister had thought the trial was unsuccessful because of "improper management," not because of the carbolic acid per se.

163 *"as if all the noises"*: David Masson, *Memories of London in the Forties* (Edinburgh: William Blackwood & Sons, 1908), 21.

166 *"cutting into the ulnar side"*: Lister, "On a New Method of Treating Compound Fracture," 329.

167 *He developed hospital gangrene*: Ibid., 357–59.

167 *"Some days later"*: Ibid., 389.

167 *Of ten compound fractures*: Fisher, *Joseph Lister*, 145.

168 *Over the coming months, Lister developed*: Ibid., 142–43.

168 *"[The] course run by cases of abscess"*: Quoted in Godlee, *Lord Lister*, 189.

169 *"I have been sometimes thinking lately"*: Ibid.

169 *Lister returned to experimenting*: Ibid., 196–97.

169 *"I now perform an operation"*: Ibid., 198.

170 *"minute particles suspended"*: Lister, "On a New Method of Treating Compound Fracture," 327.

170 *Lister's system involved using*: Michael Worboys, "Joseph Lister and the Performance of Antiseptic Surgery," *Notes and Records of the Royal Society of London* 67, no. 3 (2013), 199–209.

170 *"[The] benefits which attend this practice"*: Joseph Lister, "Illustrations of the Antiseptic System of Treatment in Surgery," *The Lancet*, Nov. 30, 1867, 668.

9. THE STORM

173 *"Medical disputes . . . are the inevitable"*: Jean-Baptiste Bouillaud, *Essai sur la philosophie médicale et sur les généralités de la clinique médicale* (Paris: Rouvier et le Bouvier, 1836), 215; translation quoted in Ann F. La Berge, "Debate as Scientific Practice in Nineteenth-Century Paris: The Controversy over the Microscope," *Perspectives on Science* 12, no. 4 (2004): 424.

174 *"All that is locally wrong"*: Sir James Paget, "The Morton Lecture on Cancer and Cancerous Diseases," *British Medical Journal*, Nov. 19, 1887, 1094.

174 *"Then came a gash"*: Lucy G. Thurston, *Life and Times of Mrs. G. Thurston* (Ann Arbor, Mich.: Andrews, 1882), 168–72, quoted in William S. Middleton, "Early Medical Experiences in Hawaii," *Bulletin of the History of Medicine* 45, no. 5 (1971): 458.

176 *"B. seems to have"*: Quoted in Godlee, *Lord Lister*, 213.

176 *"Considering* what *the operation"*: Ibid.

176 *"No one can say"*: Ibid.

176 *"I felt his true kindness"*: Ibid.

176 *"I suppose before this reaches thee"*: Ibid.

177 *Lister covered her chest*: Joseph Lister, "On Recent Improvements in the Details of Antiseptic Surgery," *The Lancet*, March 13, 1875, 366. This is a description not of Isabella's operation, but of another operation that Lister performed. It is safe to assume he followed a similar protocol with his sister.

178 *His assistant Hector Cameron*: Cameron, *Reminiscences of Lister*, 32.

178 *"I am very glad"*: Quoted in Godlee, *Lord Lister*, 213.

178 *On August 9, 1867*: Joseph Lister, "On the Antiseptic Principle in the Practice of Surgery," *British Medical Journal*, Sept. 21, 1867, 246–48.

178 *Syme had thrown his support*: James Syme, "On the Treatment of Incised Wounds with a View to Union by the First Intention," *The Lancet*, July 6, 1867, 5–6.

179 *"If Professor Lister's conclusions"*: James G. Wakley, "The Surgical Use of Carbolic Acid," *The Lancet*, Aug. 24, 1867, 234.

179 *"calculated to bring down"*: Quoted in Godlee, *Lord Lister*, 201–202.

180 *"To Professor Lister is due"*: James G. Wakley, "Carbolic Acid," *The Lancet*, Sept. 28, 1867, 410.

180 *"strange and inexplicable" use*: Quoted in Fisher, *Joseph Lister*, 152.

180 *"Nothing, he thought, should be tolerated"*: Ibid., 151.

181 *"hardly surprising"*: Joseph Lister, "On the Use of Carbolic Acid," *The Lancet*, Oct. 5, 1867, 444.

181 *The seven-hundred-page volume*: Fisher, *Joseph Lister*, 151.

181 *"I find reason to believe"*: Quoted in Godlee, *Lord Lister*, 206.

182 *"The success which has attended"*: Joseph Lister, "Carbolic Acid," *The Lancet*, Oct. 19, 1867, 502.

182 *"no difficulty in distinguishing"*: Ibid.

182 *Simpson didn't like to be challenged*: James Y. Simpson, "Carbolic Acid and Its Compounds in Surgery," *The Lancet*, Nov. 2, 1867, 548–49.

183 *"As I have already endeavoured"*: Joseph Lister, "Carbolic Acid," *The Lancet*, Nov. 9, 1867, 595.

183 *"it would be a great blessing"*: William Pirrie, "On the Use of Carbolic Acid in Burns," *The Lancet*, Nov. 9, 1867, 575.

183 *"I have always felt"*: Quoted in Godlee, *Lord Lister*, 205.

184 *"simple, effectual, and elegant"*: Frederick W. Ricketts, "On the Use of Carbolic Acid," *The Lancet*, Nov. 16, 1867, 614.

184 *"certainly not superior"*: James Morton, "Carbolic Acid: Its Therapeutic Position, with Special Reference to Its Use in Severe Surgical Cases," *The Lancet*, Feb. 5, 1870, 188.

184 *"an antiseptic mode of dressing"*: James Morton, "Carbolic Acid: Its Therapeutic Position, with Special Reference to Its Use in Severe Surgical Cases," *The Lancet*, Jan. 29, 1870, 155.

184 *In the midst of this debate*: Joseph Lister, "An Address on the Antiseptic System of Treatment in Surgery, Delivered Before the Medico-Chirurgical Society of Glasgow," *British Medical Journal* (1868): 53–56, 101–2, 461–63, 515–17; Joseph Lister, "Remarks on the Antiseptic System of Treatment in Surgery," *British Medical Journal*, April 3, 1869, 301–304.

185 *"Nature is here regarded"*: Morton, "Carbolic Acid, 155.

185 *"septic elements contained in the air"*: James G. Wakley, "Antiseptic Surgery," *The Lancet*, Oct. 29, 1870, 613.

185 *"Mr. Rouse has occasionally sponged"*: "The Use of Carbolic Acid," *The Lancet*, Nov. 14, 1868: 634.

185 *Similarly, Mr. Holmes Coote*: *The Lancet*, Dec. 5, 1868, 728.

185 *"Yet in regard to"*: "Carbolic Acid Treatment of Suppurating and Sloughing Wounds and Sores," *The Lancet*, Dec. 12, 1868, 762.

186 *In his first published article*: Gaw, "Time to Heal," 38–39.

186 *"if not with all the skill"*: James Paget, "Clinical Lecture on the Treatment of Fractures of the Leg," *The Lancet*, March 6, 1869, 317.

186 *"Are the conditions of suppuration"*: "Compound Comminuted Fracture of the Femur Without a Trace of Suppuration," *The Lancet*, Sept. 5, 1868, 324.

10. THE GLASS GARDEN

187 *"New opinions are always"*: John Locke, *Essay Concerning Human Understanding* (1690), ed. and intro. Peter H. Nidditch (Oxford, U.K.: Clarendon Press, 1975), Epistle Dedicatory, 4.

188 *"Although I was anxiously"*: The account by Annandale is reported in Robert Paterson, *Memorials of the Life of James Syme* (Edinburgh: Edmonston and Douglas, 1874), 304–305.

189 *"strong hopes are entertained"*: "Professor Syme," *The Lancet*, April 10, 1869, 506.

189 *"We only echo the feeling"*: "Professor Syme," *The Lancet*, April 17, 1869, 541.

189 *That summer, he resigned his position*: Fisher, *Joseph Lister*, 167; Godlee, *Lord Lister*, 241.

189 *"We take this step"*: Quoted in Godlee, *Lord Lister*, 242.

190 *"great happiness to all"*: Ibid.

190 *"We have throughout strongly supported"*: "The Appointment of Mr. Lister," *The Lancet*, Aug. 21, 1869, 277.

190 *Many within the medical community*: Gaw, "Time to Heal," 42.

190 *He was already aware*: Fisher, *Joseph Lister*, 165.

191 *"the latest toy of medical science"*: Donald Campbell Black, "Mr. Nunneley and the Antiseptic Treatment (Carbolic Acid)," *British Medical Journal*, Sept. 4, 1869, 281, quoted in Gaw, "Time to Heal," 46.

191 *There were similar mortality rates*: Donald Campbell Black, "Antiseptic Treatment," *The Lancet*, Oct. 9, 1869, 524–25.

192 *"To suppose that the kind"*: Joseph Lister, "Glasgow Infirmary and the Antiseptic Treatment," *The Lancet*, Feb. 5, 1870, 211.

192 *"I engaged in a perpetual contest"*: Joseph Lister, "On the Effects of the Antiseptic System of Treatment upon the Salubrity of a Surgical Hospital," *The Lancet*, Jan. 1, 1870, 4.

192 *"would hardly enter the mind"*: Lister, "Glasgow Infirmary," 211.

192 *"so far as they relate"*: Henry Lamond, "Professor Lister and the Glasgow Infirmary," *The Lancet*, Jan. 29, 1870, 175.

193 *"unsupported fancies"*: Thomas Nunneley, "Address in Surgery," *British Medical Journal*, Aug. 7, 1869, 152, 155–56.

193 *"That he should dogmatically oppose"*: Joseph Lister, "Mr. Nunneley and the Antiseptic Treatment," *British Medical Journal*, Aug. 28, 1869, 256–57.

193 *"However slowly & imperfectly the improvements"*: Joseph Jackson Lister to Joseph Lister, June 6, 1869, MS 6965/67, Wellcome Library.

194 *"prepared to see so great a change"*: Arthur Lister to Joseph Lister, Oct. 19, 1869, MS 6966/33, Wellcome Library.

194 *"He shook me warmly"*: Quoted in Godlee, *Lord Lister*, 244.

195 *"We may all rejoice"*: Joseph Lister, *Introductory lecture delivered in the University of Edinburgh*, November 8, 1869 (Edinburgh: Edmonston and Douglas, 1869), 4.

195 *"In Mr. Syme there dies"*: "[Mr Syme]," *The Lancet*, July 2, 1870, 22.

195 *"There can be no hesitation"*: "James Syme, F.R.S.E., D.C.L., Etc.," *British Medical Journal*, July 2, 1870, 25.

196 *"A new and great scientific discovery"*: Cameron, *Joseph Lister*, 100.

196 *"facts were so clear"*: F. Le M. Grasett, "Reminiscences of 'the Chief,'" in *Joseph, Baron Lister: Centenary Volume, 1827–1927*, ed. A. Logan Turner (Edinburgh: Oliver and Boyd, 1927), 109.

196 *"very dreary performances"*: Cheyne, *Lister and His Achievement*, 24.

197 *"Anything that leads a man"*: Ibid.

197 *"I have all the entrances"*: Quoted in Crowther and Dupree, *Medical Lives in the Age of Surgical Revolution*, 102.

197 *"[A] pin-drop could be heard"*: Martin Goldman, *Lister Ward* (Bristol: Adam Hilger, 1987), 61, 62.

198 *"The patients were amazed"*: Ibid., 70.

199 *just the beginning of his work*: Worboys, "Joseph Lister and the Performance of Antiseptic Surgery," 206.

200 *The opportunity soon presented itself*: See Joseph Lister, "Observations on Ligature of Arteries on the Antiseptic System," *The Lancet*,

April 3, 1869, 451–55. See also T. Gibson, "Evolution of Catgut Ligatures: The Endeavours and Success of Joseph Lister and William Macewen," *British Journal of Surgery* 77 (1990): 824–25.

200 *"I have a vivid recollection"*: Godlee, *Lord Lister*, 231.

201 *"far more than a mere contribution"*: "Professor Lister's Latest Observations," *The Lancet*, April 10, 1869, 503.

201 *Indeed, his obsession with improving*: Lister's Commonplace Books, MS0021/4/4 (9), Royal College of Surgeons of England.

202 *"Once a hospital has become"*: Erichsen, *On Hospitalism and the Causes of Death After Operations*, 98.

202 *Initially, his antiseptic system*: Joseph Lister, "A Method of Antiseptic Treatment Applicable to Wounded Soldiers in the Present War," *British Medical Journal*, Sept. 3, 1870, 243–44.

202 *"It may seem strange"*: Lister, "Further Evidence Regarding the Effects of the Antiseptic System of Treatment upon the Salubrity of a Surgical Hospital," 287–88.

202 *Those who dared to undertake*: See Stanley, *For Fear of Pain*, 89.

203 *"exactly as I have seen"*: Thomas Keith, "Antiseptic Treatment," *The Lancet*, Oct. 9, 1869, 336.

203 *"an immense step"*: E. R. Bickersteth, "Remarks on the Antiseptic Treatment of Wounds," *The Lancet*, May 29, 1869, 743.

203 *The report prompted the editor*: James G. Wakley, "Hospitalism and the Antiseptic System," *The Lancet*, Jan. 15, 1870, 91.

204 *Back in Edinburgh, John Rudd Leeson*: Account taken from Leeson, *Lister as I Knew Him*, 21–24.

11. THE QUEEN'S ABSCESS

207 *"Truth from his lips prevailed"*: Oliver Goldsmith, *The Deserted Village, A Poem*, 2nd ed. (London: W. Griffin, 1770), 10 (ll. 179–80).

208 *"arm [is] no better"*: "Journal Entry: Tuesday 29th August 1871," *Queen Victoria's Journals* 60:221, http://www.queenvictoriasjournals.org/home.do.

208 *He spoke in amazement*: Jonathan Hutchinson, "Dust and Disease," *British Medical Journal*, Jan. 29, 1879, 118–19.

209 *"citizens of Edinburgh"*: Cameron, *Joseph Lister*, 88.

210 *"I felt dreadfully nervous"*: "Journal Entry: Monday 4th September 1871,"

Queen Victoria's Journals 60:224, http://www.queenvictoriasjournals .org/home.do.

211 *"rejoiced to find nothing escape"*: Quoted in Godlee, *Lord Lister*, 305.

211 *Lister himself later claimed*: Lister later claimed that the first time he used a rubber drainage tube was on Queen Victoria. However, there's evidence in a letter between Lister and his father that he was using it as early as 1869, two years before he operated on the queen. It's possible that Lister meant that this was the first instance in which he used the rubber drainage tube in an abscess. Joseph Jackson Lister to Joseph Lister, Jan. 27, 1869, MS 6965/63, Wellcome Library. See also Lord Lister, "Remarks on Some Points in the History of Antiseptic Surgery," *The Lancet*, June 27, 1908, 1815.

211 *"Gentlemen, I am the only man"*: Quoted in Fisher, *Joseph Lister*, 194.

212 *The two men began a lengthy correspondence*: F. N. L. Pointer, "The Contemporary Scientific Background of Lister's Achievement," *British Journal of Surgery* 54 (1967): 412.

212 *"I am extremely surprised"*: Quoted in Cameron, *Joseph Lister*, 105.

212 *He traveled around the country*: For instance, Lister addressed the British Medical Association in Plymouth in 1871.

213 *"conspicuous for the small amount"*: James G. Wakley, "A Mirror of the Practice of Medicine and Surgery in the Hospitals in London," *The Lancet*, Jan. 14, 1871, 47–48.

213 *"shut out Mr. Lister's germs"*: Cameron, *Joseph Lister*, 99.

213 *"The truth is"*: Flaneur, "Antiseptic Surgery," *The Lancet*, Jan. 5, 1878, 36.

213 *"If I turn to London"*: Cameron, *Joseph Lister*, 110–11.

214 *"Man, but ye hae made"*: Quoted in Fisher, *Joseph Lister*, 159.

214 "he did not think": Quoted ibid.

217 *Lister's invitation to speak*: For the reconstruction of Lister's little-known trip through America, I am hugely indebted to Ira Rutkow's article "Joseph Lister and His 1876 Tour of America," *Annals of Surgery* 257, no. 6 (2013): 1181–87. Many of the primary sources quoted in this section were mined from his excellent article.

218 *"At the end of four weeks"*: George Derby, "Carbolic Acid in Surgery," *The Boston Medical and Surgical Journal*, Oct. 31, 1867, 273.

218 *"Mr. Lyster [sic], a surgeon"*: Ibid., 272. It's unclear why Derby misspelled Lister's name.

218 *"The wounds," explained Gay*: R. Lincoln, "Cases of Compound Fracture at the Massachusetts General Hospital Service of G. H. Gay, M.D.," *The Boston Medical and Surgical Journal*, n.s., 1, no. 10 (1868): 146.

219 *One physician from New York noted*: Quoted in John Ashhurst, ed., *Transactions of the International Medical Congress of Philadelphia, 1876* (Philadelphia: Printed for the Congress, 1877), 1028.

220 *"Is it not to be feared"*: Ibid., 532.

220 *"A large portion of American surgeons"*: Ibid.

220 *"American physicians are renowned"*: Ibid., 517, 538.

220 *One attendee accused him*: G. Shrady, "The New York Hospital," *Medical Record* 13 (1878): 113.

220–21 *"The hour being late"*: Quoted in Ashhurst, *Transactions*, 42.

221 *"Little, if any faith"*: E. H. Clarke et al., *A Century of American Medicine, 1776–1876* (Philadelphia: Henry C. Lea, 1876), 213.

221 *In Chicago, Lister's host*: Fisher, *Joseph Lister*, 223.

222 *"For me it changed surgery"*: Quoted in James M. Edmonson, *American Surgical Instruments: The History of Their Manufacture and a Directory of Instrument Makers to 1900* (San Francisco: Norman, 1997), 71.

222 *"I had no idea"*: Joseph Lister, "The Antiseptic Method of Dressing Open Wounds," *Medical Record* 11 (1876): 695–96.

222 *Lister's lecture was recorded*: Some historians have said that Lister's lecture was recorded live on a phonograph. However, the phonograph was not invented until the following year.

223 *"I have learned that the duty"*: Henry Jacob Bigelow, "Two Lectures on the Modern Art of Promoting the Repair of Tissue," *The Boston Medical and Surgical Journal*, June 5, 1879: 769–70.

224 *"We eagerly seize this occasion"*: Wrench, *Lord Lister*, 267–70.

225 *"the rules of decency"*: James G. Wakley, "Professor Lister," *The Lancet*, March 10, 1877, 361.

225 *"it would be a great benefit"*: Quoted in Fisher, *Joseph Lister*, 230.

EPILOGUE: THE DARK CURTAIN, RAISED

227 *"It is Surgery that"*: Richard Selzer, *Letters to a Young Doctor* (New York: Simon & Schuster, 1982), 51.

228 *"The impairment of my speech"*: Pasteur to Lister, Jan. 3, 1889, MS 6970/13 (in French), Wellcome Library.

228 *"You have changed Surgery"*: Nuland, *Doctors*, 380.

229 *"like the living picture"*: Quoted in Fisher, *Joseph Lister*, 294.

230 *Nothing would have come of Listerine*: Leon Morgenstern, "Gargling with Lister," *Journal of the American College of Surgeons* 204 (2007): 495–97.

232 *"Large hospitals were being abandoned"*: Wrench, *Lord Lister*, 137.

233 *In his will*: Contemporary copies of the will and codicil, MS 6979/18/1-2, Wellcome Library, found in Richard K. Aspin, "Illustrations from the Wellcome Institute Library, Seeking Lister in the Wellcome Collections," *Medical History* 41 (1997): 86–93.

234 *Henceforth, the ascendancy of knowledge*: Thomas Schlich, "Farmer to Industrialist: Lister's Antisepsis and the Making of Modern Surgery in Germany," *Notes and Records of the Royal Society* 67 (2013): 245.

234 *No longer lauded*: See Worboys, *Spreading Germs*, 24.

234 *"We knew we were in contact"*: R. H. Murray, *Science and Scientists in the Nineteenth Century* (London: Sheldon Press, 1925), 262.

ACKNOWLEDGMENTS

DIFFICULT ROADS OFTEN LEAD TO beautiful destinations. The idea for *The Butchering Art* came to me at a very low point in my life. Had it not been for the wonderful people who encouraged me to persevere even when I felt like giving up, it's unlikely this book would have ever seen the light of day.

First and foremost, I would like to offer sincere thanks to my family. To my father, Michael Fitzharris, who always believed that I was a writer even when I didn't believe it myself. And to my mother, Debbie Klebe, whose countless sacrifices throughout my childhood helped me get to where I am today. I'd also like to thank my brother, Chris Fitzharris; my stepparents, Susan Fitzharris and Greg Klebe; and my wonderful in-laws, Graham and Sandra Teal.

Thanks also to my cousins who have been like sisters to me: Lauren Pearce, Amy Martel, and Elizabeth Wilbanks. Remember, "you belong to me!"

No matter how talented a writer may be, she is nothing without someone to champion her work. Special thanks go to my agent, Anna Sproul-Latimer at the Ross-Yoon Agency, who never abandoned hope that I would someday write a book. I promise not to make you wait as long for my second project as you did for my first. I would also like to thank Hilary Knight, who is not only an amazing talent agent, but also a dear friend.

I would especially like to thank Amanda Moon, my editor at FSG, who helped me take a little story about a Victorian surgeon and turn it into an epic tale about a transformative moment in history. Your insight and acuity are second to none. Thanks also to my brilliant research assistant, Caroline Overy, whose tireless work in the archives around London helped bring color to Lister's story. And to Professor Michael Worboys, whose historical insights and feedback were invaluable while I was writing this book.

There are not many writers who would mention their divorce lawyer in the acknowledgments, but mine deserves special recognition. Farhana Shahzady fought fiercely for my rights. Thank you for teaching me to value myself again.

I am lucky to have the support of an amazing community in the form of the Order of the Good Death. Thank you to Caitlin Doughty, our fearless leader, who has been an inspiration to me, both as a person and as a writer. And to Megan Rosenbloom and Sarah Chavez

Troop, whose friendships nourish my soul. Also to Jeff Jorgensen for listening to all those late-night calls, and for believing my future could be better.

Thanks especially to Paul Koudounaris, who has always guided me wisely during pivotal moments in my life. My world is a better (and stranger) place with you in it.

There are people who have come into my life and changed its trajectory for the better. Alex Anstey crash-landed into my world many years ago. Had it not been for his creative enthusiasm, I might never have started my blog, *The Chirurgeon's Apprentice*. Thank you for being such an amazing and endless source of inspiration for me.

A heartfelt thanks goes to Dr. Bill MacLehose, friend and fellow scholar. I have admired you from the moment we met. I hope there are many more "strange drinks" and fascinating conversations in our future.

I'd like to thank those of my friends who reminded me not to let my struggle become my identity. To Shannon Marie Harmon: You are the hard shell to my taco filling. And Erica Lilly: I can always count on you to be there with tiffin when I need a pick-me-up. To Jai Virdi, whose life parallels my own in so many ways: Thank you for reminding me that giving up is never an option. I'm especially grateful to Eric Michael Johnson, who encouraged me to believe in myself as a writer. And to Jillian Drujon, without whom this book would have been finished a lot earlier. Here's to drinking too much and staying out too late.

A special thanks to my Yankee cheerleaders, Erin Reschke, Julie Cullen, Kristen Schultz, and Blair Townsend. To Shelley Estes— dreams do come true when you take a chance and choose adventure! And to the dynamic duo, Carolyn Breit and Cedric Damour. I know I can always count on you both when times get tough.

I am particularly grateful to Lori Korngiebel, whose optimism and compassion are a daily inspiration. An ocean may separate us, but we are never far apart, my soul sister. And to Edward Brooke-Hitching, Rebecca Rideal, and Dr. Joanne Paul, not only brilliant writers, but also wonderful friends. Thanks also to Sam Smith, whom I can always count on for support. Your belief in me all these years has helped me become the person I am today.

A very special thanks goes to Chris Skaife, the Ravenmaster at the Tower of London, and his beautiful wife, Jasmin, and daughter, Mickayla. Your love and encouragement have meant more to me than you could ever know. Chris, you're next!

There are people in my life who stood by me even when doing so jeopardized old friendships. To Craig Hill, whose heart is pure gold. I am your loyal friend, forever. Thanks also to Greg Walker and Thomas Waite. Your kindness and compassion helped me through some of the darkest days of my life, and I will never forget it.

People come and go, but there are some who have been there from the very beginning. Thank you to my childhood friends who stuck with me, even during my embarrassing "vampire phase"! To Marla Ginex, Alyssa Voightmann, and Kim Malinowski—thanks for all the love and laughter. I know that no matter where life takes us, we will always have one another.

I would be remiss if I did not mention the many teachers in my life who encouraged and inspired me along the way. Here I would like to thank my fifth-grade teacher, Jeff Golob, as well as my high school English teacher Barb Fryzel. I'd also like to thank Dr. Margaret Pelling, my Ph.D. supervisor at Oxford University, who continues to be an endless source of knowledge and advice. I'd especially like to thank Dr. Michael Young, who long ago introduced me to the history of science and medicine when I was an undergraduate at Illinois Wesleyan University. Had you realized I was a freshman in your senior class, my life may have turned out differently! Thank you for your friendship and support.

And last but certainly not least, I would like to thank my wonderful husband, Adrian Teal. It is not too much to say that I would be lost without you. Each day we have together is a blessing. I look forward to a bright and happy future by your side. I love you.

INDEX

amputations, 3, 10–15, 84, 90–91,
98, 180; antiseptic treatment of
compound fractures versus,
163–65, 167; battlefield, 110–11,
219; ligatures for, 91, 180, 199;
mortality rates for, 55, 143, 191,
203; prosthetics for survivors of,
77; surgical tools for, 10–12,
14–15, 17, 31–33, 90, 219;
see also stumps

anatomical studies, 29, 30, 49, 79,
94–96, 133, 146; comparative,
86–87; microscopic, 34, 133, 205

anatomical theaters, 4, 45

anatomizations, *see* dissections

Anderson, Thomas, 149, 155, 162

Andral, Gabriel, 34

anesthetics, *see* chloroform; ether

Anglican church, 26

animals, experiments on, 124–26

Annandale, Thomas, 187, 188

antiseptic system, 161, 171, 197,
202, 215, 217, 225, 234, 253*n*;
American response to, 219–21;
Pasteur's influence on
development of, 159–60;
spontaneous generation theory
refuted by, 52, 198; *see also*
carbolic acid

apothecaries, 9

Appleton, Martha, 73

Arlidge, John Thomas, 73

Arnott, Neil, 54

arsenic, 26, 44

arteries, tying off, *see* ligatures

artificial insemination, 80–81

Asma, Stephen, 243*n*

atropine, 43

Australia, 69, 70

bacteria, 47, 52, 64, 121, 156–57,
198, 208–209; chemicals for

destruction of, *see* antiseptics;
dissection and exposure to, 41,
50; surgical instruments as
havens for, 32; *see also* germ
theory; infections, bacterial

Balfour, Isaac Bayley, 224

Ballingall, George, 110

Balmoral Castle (Scotland), 207,
210, 211

Barnum, P. T., 49, 243*n*

Beddoe, John, 106–107

Bell, Alexander Graham, 217

Bell, Charles, 14

Bell, John, 82, 83

Berlioz, Hector, 39

Bible, 43

Bichat, Marie François Xavier, 34

Bickersteth, E. R., 203

Bigelow, Henry Jacob, 7–8, 41,
218, 222–23

Bigelow, Jacob, 41

Bigo (wine merchant), 155, 156

biochemistry, 156, 247*n*

Black, Donald Campbell, 191, 203

Blackwell's Island Charity Hospital
(New York), 221–22

bladder stones, 12

Blockley Almshouse
(Philadelphia), 52

blood coagulation, 135, 142

bloodletting, 32

blood poisoning, *see* septicemia

Bloomsbury (London), 26

body snatchers, 95–96

Bonaparte, Prince Jérôme, 16

bone saws, 10–11, 14–15, 31–33,
90, 219

Boott, Francis, 8

Boston, 222–23

Boston Medical and Surgical Journal,
8, 218

Boston Society for Medical
Improvement, 218

Gross Clinic, The (Eakins), 217, 232
Grove House boarding school, 29–30
Guthrie, Douglas, 140
Guthrie, George James, 65
Guy, William Augustus, 31
Guy's Hospital (London), 62, 86, 151

Hair, Philip, 182
Halle (Germany), 202
Hamilton, Frank, 220
Hard, Addison Davis, 80–81
Hare, William, 94
Harper's New Monthly Magazine, 40
Harvard University, 41, 146, 217, 223
hemorrhages, 47, 91, 103, 117, 139, 167
Henley, W. E., 105
hepatitis, 86
hernias, 64–65
HMS *Saturn* (ship), 83
Hodgkin, John, 29–30, 42–44
Hodgkin, Thomas, 29
Holmes, Oliver Wendell, 146
homeopathic medicine, 52
homeopathy, 134
Hooke, Robert, 125
hospitalism, 53–55, 82, 142, 145, 152
house surgeons: Lister's, 139–41, 148, 165, 214; Erichsen's, 51, 71, 85, 86; Syme's, 100, 103–105, 114, 190
Hunter, William, 89
Hutton, James, 106

Ilfracombe (England), 44
Illustrated London News, 77
industrial accidents, 72–74, 137
infant mortality, 24
infections, 6, 17, 46, 52–53, 85, 171, 194, 196; bacterial, 13, 47; of compound fractures, 163–65; dissections as source of, 50, 56; hospital, 85, 145, 155, 159, 161, 165, 177; medical students susceptible, 41; after surgery, *see* postoperative infections; venereal, 62, 74–75, 198, 222; *see also* inflammation; putrefaction; suppuration
inflammation, 13, 62, 88, 120–27, 145, 197; antiseptics to prevent and treat, 160–61, 165, 209; of bowel, *see* peritonitis; Lister's research on, 123–27, 135, 142, 253*n*
internal medicine, 17
International Medical Congress (London), 229
International Medical Congress (Philadelphia), 215, 217–23, 229, 231
International Red Cross, 104
Ireland, 44, 119; immigrants from, 93, 136
Isle of Wight (England), 44
Islington (London), 56

Jack the Ripper, 32
Jenner, William, 210
Jennings, George, 77
John Bull, 27
Johnson, Steven, 25
Johnson, William Henry, 243*n*
Johnson & Johnson, 231
Jones, Wharton, 81, 124, 126

Keen, William W., 222
Keith, Thomas, 202–203
Kelly, Matthew, 75

INDEX

Kelvin, William Thomas, Lord, 132–33

Kensal Green Cemetery (London), 50

Kidd, Captain, 67

King, Charles Glen, 247n

King's College (London), 26, 223–25, 228; Hospital, 9, 62

Kinross (Scotland), 123

knives, 5, 25, 29, 48, 72, 96; amputation, 10–12, 14, 15, 17, 32; criminal use of, 32, 59, 61–64, 69, 102; dissecting, 37, 41; household injuries caused by, 73; surgical, 31, 91–92, 140, 174, 175, 177, 198, 231

Knox, Robert, 94

Koch, Robert, 209

Kölliker, Albert von, 81

lacerations, 17

Lambert, Jordan Wheat, 230

Lamond, Henry, 192

Lancet, The, 6, 55, 160, 189, 190, 213, 215; calls for tests in London hospitals of Lister's methods, 203, 212; criticism of Lister published in, 179–86, 192, 225; Fothergillian Gold Medal competition announced in, 65–66; Lister's disinfection articles in, 169–70, 178, 198, 201, 217; Liston's obituary in, 50; Syme's obituary in, 195; Syme's report on carbolic acid treatment of compound fractures in, 178–79

lancets, 31

Larecy (painter), 73

Lawrence, Joseph Joshua, 229–30

Lawrie, James, 129–30, 135

Leach, Harvey, 48–50

lead, illness caused by exposure to, 73

leeches, 65, 66; artificial, 77

Leeds (England), 193

Leeson, John Rudd, 204–205

Lemaire, Jules, 179, 181, 182

Letheon, 8

Lewes, George Henry, 151

ligatures, 31, 65, 200–201, 203; for amputations, 15, 91, 180, 199

Lille University, 155

linseed oil, 161, 168, 177

Lister, Agnes Syme (wife), 132, 133, 143, 189, 190, 214; courtship and wedding of, 116–19; death of, 228; frog experiments assisted by, 123–24, 126; nursing of ill relatives by, 143, 189

Lister, Arthur (brother), 119, 193–94

Lister, Arthur (nephew), 233, 234

Lister, Isabella (mother), 20, 22, 52, 116–17, 133, 134, 144

Lister, Isabella (sister), *see* Pim, Isabella Lister

Lister, John (brother), 42

Lister, Joseph: accolades in later years of, 229; Agnes as research assistant to, 123–24, 126; antiseptic system developed by, 161–71, 198–205, 212–14; appointed Regius Professor, 130–31; arrival at University College London of, 23, 26, 27; artistic skill of, 22–23, 78–81, 85, 233; arts degree completed by, 27–28; birth of, 20; childhood of, 19–22, 29–30; correspondence of father and, 23, 43, 44, 101, 114, 120, 130, 143–45, 169, 176, 181, 183–84, 188, 193; death of, 233–34;

279